HANDBOOK OF
Retinal **OCT**

SECOND EDITION

HANDBOOK OF
Retinal OCT

Editors

Jay S. Duker, MD
Director, New England Eye Center
Professor and Chair, Department of
Ophthalmology
Tufts Medical Center
Tufts University School of Medicine
Boston, MA
USA

Nadia K. Waheed, MD, MPH
Professor in Ophthalmology
New England Eye Center
Tufts Medical Center
Tufts University School of Medicine
Boston, MA
USA

Darin R. Goldman, MD
Vitreo-retinal Surgeon
Partner, Retina Group of Florida
Clinical Affiliate Associate Professor of
Surgery
Charles E. Schmidt College of Medicine
Florida Atlantic University
Boca Raton, FL
USA

ELSEVIER

Elsevier
1600 John F. Kennedy Blvd.
Ste 1800
Philadelphia, PA 19103-2899

HANDBOOK OF RETINAL OCT, SECOND EDITION

ISBN: 978-0-323-75772-0

Previous edition copyrighted 2014

Library of Congress Control Number 2021939121

Senior Content Strategist: Kayla Wolfe
Senior Content Development Specialist: Angie Breckon
Publishing Services Manager: Shereen Jameel
Senior Project Manager: Karthikeyan Murthy
Design Direction: Brian Salisbury

Printed in India
Last digit is the print number: 9 8 7 6 5 4 3 2

Working together
to grow libraries in
developing countries

www.elsevier.com • www.bookaid.org

Contents

Preface ix
List of Contributors xi
Acknowledgments..xiii
Dedications xiii
Glossary xv

Part 1: Introduction to OCT 1

Section 1:   OCT: What It Is 2
    1.1   *Scanning Principles* 2
    Emily S. Levine

    1.2   *Basic Scan Patterns and OCT Output* 4
    Emily S. Levine

Section 2:   Data and Interpretation.. 10
    2.1   *OCT Interpretation* 10
    Emily S. Levine

Section 3:   OCT Artifacts.. 12
    3.1   *Artifacts on SD-OCT and OCTA*.................................... 12
    Eugenia Custo Greig

Section 4:   Normal Retinal Anatomy and Basic Pathologic Appearances .. 24
    4.1   *Normal Retinal Anatomy and Basic Pathologic Appearances* .. 24
    Emily S. Levine

Part 2: Optic Nerve Disorders 37

Section 5:   Optic Nerve Disorders 38
    5.1   *Basic Optic Nerve Scan Patterns and Output* 38
    Daniela Ferrara, Alexandre S.C. Reis, and Alessandro A. Jammal

Part 3: Macular Disorders 41

Section 6:   Dry Age-Related Macular Degeneration.................................... 42
    6.1   *Dry Age-Related Macular Degeneration* 42
Section 7:   Wet Age-Related Macular Degeneration 46
    7.1   *Wet Age-Related Macular Degeneration* 46
Section 8:   Macular Pathology Associated With Myopia 56
    8.1   *Posterior Staphyloma* 56
    8.2   *Myopic Choroidal Neovascular Membrane*.......................... 58
    8.3   *Myopic Macular Schisis* 62
    8.4   *Dome-Shaped Macula*.. 64
    8.5   *Myopic Tractional Retinal Detachment* 66
Section 9: Vitreomacular Interface Disorders 68
    9.1   *Pachychoroid Syndromes*.. 68
    Luísa S.M. Mendonça

    9.2   *Vitreomacular Adhesion and Vitreomacular Traction*.............. 74
    Omar Abu-Qamar

    9.3   *Full Thickness Macular Hole*... 78
    Emily S. Levine

    9.4   *Lamellar Macular Hole* 82
    Emily S. Levine

    9.5   *Epiretinal Membrane* 84
    Emily S. Levine

Section 10: Miscellaneous Causes of Macular Edema 88
    10.1 Postoperative Cystoid Macular Edema 88
    10.2 Macular Telangiectasia 90
    10.3 Uveitis 96
Section 11: Miscellaneous Macular Disorders 100
    11.1 Central Serous Chorioretinopathy 100
    Omar Abu-Qamar

    11.2 Hydroxychloroquine Toxicity 104
    11.3 Pattern Dystrophy 108
    11.4 Oculocutaneous Albinism 112
    11.5 Subretinal Perfluorocarbon 114
    11.6 X-Linked Juvenile Retinoschisis 116

Part 4: Vaso-Occlusive Disorders 119

Section 12: Diabetic Retinopathy 120
    12.1 Non-Proliferative Diabetic Retinopathy 120
    Omar Abu-Qamar

    12.2 Non-Proliferative Diabetic Retinopathy With Macular Edema .. 126
    Omar Abu-Qamar

    12.3 Proliferative Diabetic Retinopathy 130
    Omar Abu-Qamar

Section 13: Retinal Vein Obstruction 136
    13.1 Branch Retinal Vein Obstruction 136
    Eugenia Custo Greig

    13.2 Central Retinal Vein Obstruction 140
    Eugenia Custo Greig

Section 14: Retinal Artery Obstruction 144
    14.1 Branch Retinal Artery Obstruction 144
    14.2 Central Retinal Artery Obstruction 148
    14.3 Cilioretinal Artery Obstruction 152
    14.4 Paracentral Acute Middle Maculopathy 154

Part 5: Inherited Retinal Degenerations 159

Section 15: Inherited Retinal Degenerations 160
    15.1 Retinitis Pigmentosa 160
    15.2 Stargardt Disease 162
    15.3 Best Disease 164
    15.4 Cone Dystrophy 166

Part 6: Uveitis and Inflammatory Diseases 169

Section 16: Posterior Non-Infectious Uveitis 170
    16.1 Multifocal Choroditis 170
    Emily S. Levine

    16.2 Birdshot Chorioretinopathy 174
    Emily S. Levine

    16.3 Serpiginous Choroiditis 178
    Emily S. Levine

    16.4 Vogt–Koyanagi–Harada Disease 182
    Emily S. Levine

    16.5 Sympathetic Ophthalmia 184
    Emily S. Levine

16.6 *Posterior Scleritis* 186
Emily S. Levine

Section 17: Posterior Infection Uveitis 188
17.1 *Toxoplasma Chorioretinitis* 188
Eduardo Uchiyama

17.2 *Tuberculosis* 192
Eduardo Uchiyama

17.3 *Acute Syphilitic Posterior Placoid Chorioretinitis* 196
Eduardo Uchiyama

17.4 *Candida Albicans Endogenous Endophthalmitis* 198
Eduardo Uchiyama

17.5 *Acute Retinal Necrosis Syndrome* 200
Eduardo Uchiyama

Part 7: Trauma 203

Section 18: Physical Trauma 204
18.1 *Commotio Retinae* 204
18.2 *Choroidal Rupture and Subretinal Hemorrhage* 206
18.3 *Valsalva Retinopathy* 208
Section 19: Photothermal, Photomechanical, and Photochemical Trauma .. 210
19.1 *Laser Injury (Photothermal and Photomechanical)* 210
19.2 *Solar Maculopathy* 212

Part 8: Tumors 215

Section 20: Choroidal Tumors 216
20.1 *Choroidal Nevus* 216
20.2 *Choroidal Melanoma* 220
20.3 *Choroidal Hemangioma* 224
Section 21: Retinal Tumors 228
21.1 *Retinal Capillary Hemangioma* 228
21.2 *Retinoblastoma* 230
Section 22: Other Tumors 232
22.1 *Metastatic Choroidal Tumor* 232
22.2 *Vitreoretinal Lymphoma* 234
22.3 *Primary Uveal Lymphoma* 238

Part 9: Peripheral Retinal Abnormalities 241

Section 23: Retinal Detachment 242
23.1 *Retinal Detachment* 242
Omar Abu-Qamar

Section 24: Retinoschisis 244
24.1 *Retinoschisis* 244
Omar Abu-Qamar

Section 25: Peripheral Lattice Degeneration 248
25.1 *Peripheral Lattice Degeneration* 248
Omar Abu-Qamar

Index 251

Preface

Optical coherence tomography (OCT) was "discovered" in an optics lab at the Massachusetts Institute of Technology in the late 1980s by James Fujimoto and his collaborators: Carmen Puliafito, Joel Schuman, David Huang, Eric Swanson, and Mike Hee. It began as an effort to experimentally measure excimer laser corneal ablation in real time. While it failed in that regard, the founders quickly identified the possibility that OCT could be employed to measure static ocular tissue thickness in real time. The first publication on OCT was in *Science* in 1991, and by 1996 the technology was transferred to a commercial company, and soon thereafter commercial devices began to be sold.

It is safe to say that OCT is one of the most important ancillary tests in ophthalmology and is indisputably *the* most important ancillary test in the subspecialty of the retina. In the first edition, we set out to produce an easy-to-read, brief but complete handbook of OCT images that was disease-based. Given the importance of OCT in our practices, we concluded that the OCT images should be the major focus of the book. Consistency of chapter layout, excellent images, and well-documented pathologic features were all goals. We feel we succeeded.

The second edition carries on the format of minimal clinical description of the pathologic entities, as there are plenty of excellent textbooks that cover these entities in more depth. We have expanded the book to include a number of new pathological entities. In addition, we have added optical coherence tomography angiography (OCTA) where appropriate.

We hope you find this handbook useful in your clinical practice on a daily basis.

Jay S. Duker, MD
Nadia K. Waheed, MD, MPH
Darin R. Goldman, MD

List of Contributors

Omar Abu-Qamar, MD, MMSc
OCT Research Fellow
New England Eye Center
Tufts Medical Center
Tufts University School of Medicine
Boston, MA
USA

Eugenia Custo Greig, MD
Yale School of Medicine
New Haven, CT
USA

Daniela Ferrara, MD, MSc, PhD
Assistant Professor of Ophthalmology
Tufts University School of Medicine
Boston, MA
USA

Darin R. Goldman, MD
Vitreo-retinal Surgeon
Partner, Retina Group of Florida
Clinical Affiliate Associate Professor of Surgery
Charles E. Schmidt College of Medicine
Florida Atlantic University
Boca Raton, FL
USA

Alessandro A. Jammal, MD
Research Scientist
Duke Eye Center
Duke University
Durham, NC
USA
Glaucoma Specialist
State University of Campinas
Campinas
Brazil

Emily S. Levine, MD, MTM
Resident Physician in Ophthalmology
Dartmouth Hitchcock Medical Center
Lebanon, NH
USA

Luísa S.M. Mendonça, MD
Department of Ophthalmology
Federal University of São Paulo
São Paulo
Brazil

Alexandre S.C. Reis, MD, PhD
Unicamp
Opthalmology
Campinas
Brazil

Eduardo Uchiyama, MD
Uveitis Specialist
Vitreo-Retinal Surgeon
Retina Group of Florida
Fort Lauderdale, FL
Affiliate Assistant Professor
Charles E. Schmidt College of Medicine
Florida Atlantic University
Boca Raton, FL
USA

Nadia K. Waheed, MD, MPH
Professor in Ophthalmology
New England Eye Center
Tufts Medical Center
Tufts University School of Medicine
Boston, MA
USA

Acknowledgments

The development of optical coherence tomography and its emergence as the most important ancillary test in ophthalmology is inextricably linked to the New England Eye Center at Tufts Medical Center and its physicians. The clinical experiences summarized in this book are based on the collective expertise gained at the Eye Center over the past three decades, and we are very grateful to our colleagues Caroline Baumal, Elias Reichel, Chris Robinson, Andre Witkin, Michelle Liang, and Shilpa Desai with whom we are privileged to share patients and who have been an inexhaustible resource for this endeavor.

We would also like to acknowledge the unparalleled ophthalmic imaging department at the New England Eye Center whose members acquired most of the images included in this book. Thanks also go out to the contributing authors and to our production team at Elsevier who worked on a very tight schedule to get the book published in just over six months. Our fellows and residents, whose questions provide constant intellectual challenge, also deserve acknowledgment. And last but perhaps most importantly, we would like to thank our families for their patience and support.

Dedications

To my wife, Julie, and my children, Jake, Bear, Sam, and Elly, whose support, love, patience, and understanding allow me to pursue projects like this book. Also, to Carmen Puliafito, Joel Schuman, and Jim Fujimoto—without them OCT would not exist and without their mentorship and collaboration I would never have become immersed in it.

Jay S. Duker

To Khadija and Ahmed, for their patience, generosity, support, and encouragement. To my mother, Khalida, the constant inspiration, who set and supported me on a path that few have the good fortune to follow. None of this would be possible without the three of you. To my dad, whose grace and good humor have always been an inspiration. To my mentors past and present, and to my co-authors who made the process of writing this book such a phenomenally enjoyable and educational experience.

Nadia K. Waheed

To my wife, Robin, whose constant love and encouragement allow me to pursue my many passions. To my children, Rona, Cole, and Lexi, who keep me grounded and on my toes. To my parents, Marisse and Tony, whose support I am forever grateful to have. Lastly, to my mentors, who paved the way ahead giving me a clear path to achieve my professional aspirations.

Darin R. Goldman

Glossary

AMD age-related macular degeneration
ARN acute retinal necrosis

BM Bruch's membrane
BRAO branch retinal artery obstruction
BRVO branch retinal vein obstruction

CiRAO cilioretinal artery obstruction
CME cystoid macular edema
CNV choroidal neovascularization
CRAO central retinal artery obstruction
CRVO central retinal vein obstruction
CSCR central serous chorioretinopathy
CWS cotton wool spots

DME diabetic macular edema
DR diabetic retinopathy

EDI enhanced depth imaging
ELM external limiting membrane
ERM epiretinal membrane
ETDRS Early Treatment of Diabetic Retinopathy Study

FA fluorescein angiography
FAF fundus autofluorescence
FD Fourier domain
FTMH full-thickness macular hole

GA geographic atrophy
GCC ganglion cell complex

HE hard exudates
HRVO hemiretinal vein obstruction

ICGA indocyanine green angiography
ICP intracranial pressure
ILM internal limiting membrane
INL inner nuclear layer
IPL inner plexiform layer
IRF intraretinal fluid
IRMA intraretinal microvascular abnormalities
IS inner segment of photoreceptors
IS–OS inner segment–outer segment (of photoreceptors)

LE left eye

LMH lamellar macular hole

MacTel macular telangiectasia
MCP multifocal choroiditis with panuveitis

NFL nerve fiber layer
NPDR non-proliferative diabetic retinopathy
NVD neovascularization of the disc
NVE neovascularization elsewhere (retinal neovascularization)
NVI neovascularization of the iris

OCT optical coherence tomography
ONH optic nerve head
ONL outer nuclear layer
OPL outer plexiform layer
OS outer segment of photoreceptors

PCME postoperative cystoid macular edema
PCV polypoidal choroidal vasculopathy
PDR proliferative diabetic retinopathy
PED pigment epithelial detachment
PFC perfluorocarbon
PVD posterior vitreous detachment

RAP retinal angiomatous proliferation
RCH retinal capillary hemangioma
RD retinal detachment
RE right eye
RNFL retinal nerve fiber layer
RP retinitis pigmentosa
RPE retinal pigment epithelium
RRD rhegmatogenous retinal detachment
RS retinoschisis

SD spectral domain
SD-OCT spectral domain optical coherence tomography
SRF subretinal fluid
SS swept source
SS-OCT swept source optical coherence tomography
SVP summed voxel projection

TD time domain

Glossary

TD-OCT time domain optical coherence tomography

TRD tractional retinal detachment

TSINT temporal, superior, inferior, nasal temporal scan pattern

VEGF vascular endothelial growth factor

VKH Vogt–Koyanagi–Harada

VMA vitreomacular adhesion

VMT vitreomacular traction

VRL vitreoretinal lymphoma

XLRS X-linked juvenile retinoschisis

PART 1: Introduction to OCT

Section 1: OCT: What It Is 2

1.1 *Scanning Principles* 2
Emily S. Levine

1.2 *Basic Scan Patterns and OCT Output* 4
Emily S. Levine

Section 2: Data and Interpretation 10

2.1 *OCT Interpretation* 10
Emily S. Levine

Section 3: OCT Artifacts 12

3.1 *Artifacts on SD-OCT and OCTA* 12
Eugenia Custo Greig

Section 4: Normal Retinal Anatomy and Basic Pathologic Appearances .. 24

4.1 *Normal Retinal Anatomy and Basic*
Pathologic Appearances 24
Emily S. Levine

1

1.1 Scanning principles

Optical coherence tomography (OCT) is a medical diagnostic imaging technology that captures micron resolution three-dimensional images. It is based on the principle of optical reflectometry, which involves the measurement of light back-scattering through transparent or semitransparent media such as biological tissues. It achieves this by measuring the intensity and the echo time delay of light that is scattered from the tissues of interest. Light from a broadband light source is broken into two arms, a reference arm and a sample arm that is reflected back from structures at various depths within the posterior pole of the eye.

There are two main ways in which the backscattered light can be detected:
- Time domain (TD) detection
- Fourier domain (FD) detection, which is further broken down into:
  - Spectral domain (SD)
  - Swept source (SS)

Time Domain OCT

In time domain OCT scanning, light from the reference arm and light reflected back from the sample undergo interference, and the interference over time is used to generate an A-scan depth resolved image of the retina at a single point. Moving the sample and the light source with respect to each other generates multiple A-scans that are combined into a cross-sectional linear image called the B-scan or line scan. Scanning speeds of TD-OCTs are typically around 400 A-scans/second. These older-generation machines are now rarely used in clinical practice.

Spectral Domain OCT

In this technology, the spectral interference pattern between the reference beam and the sample beam is dispersed by a spectrometer and collected simultaneously with an array detector. This simultaneous collection allows much faster scanning speeds than the traditional time domain devices where a mechanically moving interferometer gathers the data over time. An A-scan is then generated using an inverse Fourier transform on the simultaneously gathered data. Commercially available SD-OCT devices have scanning rates of 40,000–100,000 A-scans/second.

Higher scan speeds in the SD-OCT allow faster acquisition time, which minimizes the chance of eye movements during acquisition. Both hardware and software enhancements permit precise image registration, which allows for a more reliable comparison between visits. Faster acquisition speeds also mean a higher sampling density of the macula, minimizing the chances of missing pathology and allowing the production of three-dimensional OCT scans. The broader light sources of SD-OCT devices achieve a higher axial resolution than TD-OCT, providing better visualization of retinal anatomy. At present, there are eight commercial SD-OCT devices that are available in at least some, if not all, large international markets.

Swept Source OCT

In swept source (or optical frequency domain) OCT scanning, the light source is rapidly swept in wavelength and the spectral interference pattern is detected on a single or small number of receivers as a function of time. The spectral interference patterns obtained as a function of time then undergo a reverse Fourier transform to generate an A-scan image. Higher scanning speeds allow for denser sampling and better registration. Swept source OCT also has less sensitivity roll-off with depth, allowing for a better visualization of structures deep to the retina. At present, swept source OCT is not widely available commercially, with only two commercially available devices.

OCT Angiography

OCT angiography (OCTA) is an application of OCT that noninvasively visualizes the vascular layers of the retina. The microvasculature is not depicted in OCT images because it does not produce back-scatter distinct from its surrounding tissue. Instead, OCTA takes advantage of motion contrast between moving blood flow and the static retinal surroundings to visualize the vasculature. In sequentially repeated B-scans taken at the same position, the only differences, or decorrelation, in reflectivity come from sites of blood flow. Higher resolutions and scan speeds in contemporary OCT devices allow B-scans to be repeated fast enough to resolve the vasculature adequately.

OCTA devices use different algorithms to calculate motion contrast between repeated B-scans. Swept source OCTA offers less sensitivity loss with depth, which permits better visualization of the deeper vasculature of the choroid and choriocapillaris.

Each commercially available OCT device uses unique scan patterns that are programmed into the machine. There is considerable overlap between devices, however, with several general scan patterns available across all devices. The scan patterns for the major commercially available machines are summarized in Table 1.2.1. The two most commonly used scans in evaluating retinal disease are:

▸ Macular cube scan
▸ Line scan(s)

Depending on the particular machine, scan patterns may be programmable with respect to functions such as pixel density, B-scan density, speed, ability to oversample, and length of scanned image.

Macular Cube Scan

Cube scans are volume or 3D scans analogous to computed tomography or magnetic resonance scans that acquire volumetric cubes of data. SD-OCT machines acquire a rapid series of line scans (B-scans), typically in a 6 mm × 6 mm square area centered on the fovea. The scans are generally at relatively low resolution to minimize the time of scanning. As a result, when examining individual line scans from a cube scan, some detail is lost. As a default, the cube scan is centered at the fovea, but other areas of interest can be captured by manually centering the scan elsewhere in the retina. Optic nerve topographic scans are cube scans centered on the nerve. Cube scans are generally used to generate 3D viewing of the OCT.

In the Zeiss Cirrus SD-OCT, there are two macular cube scans available, both capturing a 6 mm × 6 mm area, with no ability to customize. There is a faster 200 × 200 cube (200 B-scans each composed of 200 A-scans) or the slightly slower 512 × 128 cube (128 B-scans each composed of 512 A-scans) that has higher quality horizontal scans. The volume scan on the Heidelberg Spectralis uses a similar raster scanning protocol with a fast 25 B-scans each consisting of 512 sample points or A-scans or with a dense 1024 × 49 default scanning protocol. The Topcon 3D-OCT offers a 256 × 256 or 512 × 128 scanning protocol. The Optovue RT-Vue 3D Retina scan protocol yields a 74 mm × 7 mm macular cube scan with 141 B-scans consisting of 385 A-scans each.

▸ Raster Scans: raster scanning is one method used to obtain cube scans of the macula. This involves a systematic pattern of image capture over a rectangular area using closely spaced parallel lines. It leads to a uniform sampling density over the entire area being scanned with the OCT.

▸ Radial Scans: these consist of 6 to 18 high-resolution line scans taken at radial orientations, all passing through the fovea. The Optovue RT-Vue's radial scan pattern consists of 18 lines radially oriented to the fovea, which can be adjusted to be between 2 and 12 mm in length. The Heidelberg Spectralis has a 6-line macular radial scan and the Topcon 3D-OCT Maestro has a 12-line radial scan. A disadvantage of the radial line scans is that the machine interpolates between the scans when generating macular thickness maps. This is reasonable for the fovea where the lines are close to each other, but it can miss lesions further out in the macula where the lines are spaced further apart.

TABLE 1.2.1 SCAN PATTERNS IN COMMONLY USED OCT DEVICES

	Zeiss Cirrus	Heidelberg Spectralis	Optovue RT-Vue	Topcon 3-D OCT Maestro	Canon Xephilio OCT-A1	Nidek OCT RS-3000	Bioptogen SD-OCT
3D scans	Macular cube	Volume scan	3D Retina 3D Widefield	3D Macula	Macula 3D Multi-cross	Macula map	Rectangular volume Mixed volume
Line scans	1-line raster scan 5-line raster scan 21-line raster scan cross	7-line raster scan	Line scan HD Line Raster Cross-line HD cross-Line	Line 5-Line Cross	Cross	Macula multi Macula line	Linear scan
Radial scans	Radial	No presets, can be selected	Radial Lines	Radial		Macula radial	Radial volume
Mesh scan	None *		Grid			Macula multi	

▸ Mesh Scans: Some machines include a mesh or grid scanning pattern that acquires vertical and horizontal B-scans over the area of interest. The grid protocol of the RT-Vue consists of five vertical lines and five horizontal lines, and the total pattern can be adjusted to be between 2 and 12 mm in length and 0–8 mm wide.

Line, Cross-Line and Raster Scans

Line scans are a single B-scan composed of generally a higher number of A-scans than the cube scans. This higher sampling density allows higher-resolution scans of the retinal tissue to be acquired. In addition, oversampling can be performed to increase signal-noise ratio (Fig. 1.2.1). The Cirrus five-line raster consists of five horizontal 3, 6, or 9-mm lines each scanned four times and averaged. The 5 lines in the raster can be collapsed to obtain a single line scan that consists of 20 averaged B-scans (Fig. 1.2.2). The RT-Vue raster scan consists of 21 parallel line scans that can be adjusted to be between 6 and 12 mm in length and 1–8 mm wide. The seven-line raster of the Heidelberg also spans a 6 mm × 6 mm area of the macula. Heidelberg can be programmed to oversample a line scan up to 100 times at each point.

Widefield Scans

Widefield scans encompass a region of the retina larger than the typical 6 mm × 6 mm macular cubes or line scans, often including both the macula and the disc. Swept source OCT (SS-OCT) allows for wider scanning of the posterior pole. The Zeiss PLEX Elite 9000 SS-OCT performs three 12 mm × 12 mm macular cubes, with a 512 × 512, an 800 × 800, and a 1024 × 1024 scan protocol. The swept source Topcon device generates 12 mm × 9 mm widefield OCT scans. The newest version of the Topcon SD-OCT also offers widefield 12 mm × 9 mm scans.

Enhanced Depth Imaging

Enhanced depth imaging (EDI) protocols, now available in all major commercial OCT devices, use a combination of image averaging and moving the zero delay line of the SD-OCT closer to the choroid to obtain higher-resolution images of the choroid. EDI is invaluable in diseases that involve the choroid where somewhat higher choroidal resolution is needed, as well as diseases with choroidal thickening where the sclerochoroidal border may not be visible on standard scanning protocols.

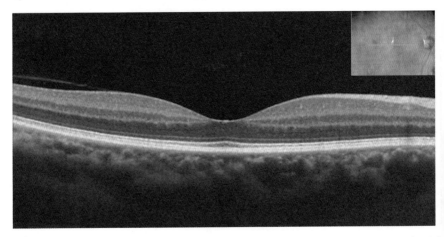

Figure 1.2.1 Line scan through the macula. Inset depicts an *en face* image of the summoned voxel projection with a cyan line indicating the location of the line scan.

Macular Maps

Macular maps are derived directly from either the cube scan data or radial scans, depending on the machine. They come in two forms:

▸ numeric displays showing the average retinal thickness in the zone of interest
▸ color-coded displays illustrating the difference between the examination and age-matched normative data base (Fig. 1.2.3).

C-Scans (*En Face* Images), OCT Fundus Image (Rendered Fundus Image, Summed Voxel Projection [SVP])

This image resembles a red-free image of the retina and is obtained by summation of data from all the B-scans. It is currently available in all SD-OCT machines except Heidelberg (Fig. 1.2.1, inset).

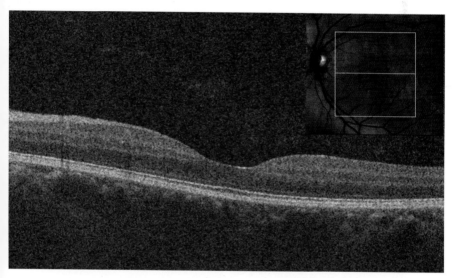

Figure 1.2.2 Single B-scan from a macular cube, with the inset depicting the location of the B-scan. Note the lower resolution of the B-scan in comparison with the line scan in Figure 1.2.1.

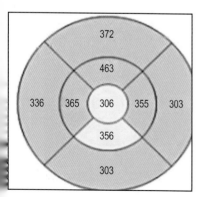

Figure 1.2.3 Macular map showing retinal thickness.

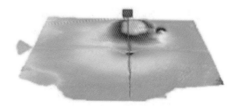

Figure 1.2.4 Topographical map.

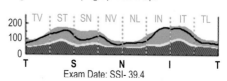

Figure 1.2.5 Retinal nerve fiber layer analysis.

Topographical Maps

Retinal thickness data obtained from segmented 3D datasets are used to form a 2D topographical data set that can be displayed in false color (color-coded) displays or as an overlay on the OCT-rendered fundus image to obtain a quick topographic picture of the macula, internal limiting membrane, or retinal pigment epithelium layer (Fig. 1.2.4).

Nerve Fiber Layer Map

Segmented 3D datasets over the optic nerve can be used to generate nerve fiber layer thickness measurements that can then be compared with age-matched controls and displayed in a color-coded pattern (Fig. 1.2.5).

Optical Coherence Tomography Angiography (OCTA)

Scan patterns used to generate OCTA images are generally cubes that are 3 mm × 3 mm or 6 mm × 6 mm in size centered on the fovea or the optic nerve. SS-OCTA devices can produce wider field scans such as a 12 mm × 12 mm scan or even a 15 mm × 9 mm scan in a single acquisition. Additionally, both SD-OCTA and SS-OCTA scans can achieve a wider field of view by automatically montaging multiple acquisitions, a feature that is currently available in both the Optovue and the Zeiss Plex Elite Devices (Fig. 1.2.6).

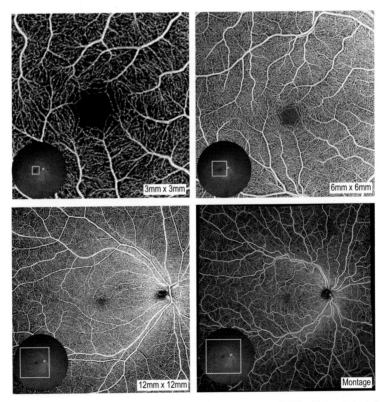

Figure 1.2.6 *En face* OCTA images of the superficial capillary plexus (SCP) with inset depicting the scan area (clockwise from top left: 3 mm × 3 mm, 6 mm × 6 mm, 12 mm × 12 mm, and a montage of multiple 12 mm × 12 mm images).

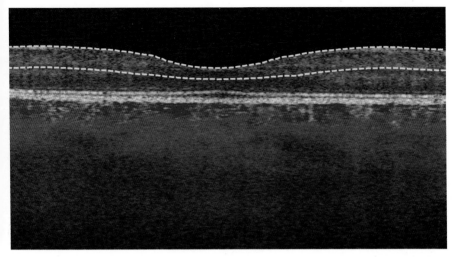

Figure 1.2.7 Line scan through the macula with flow signal overlay in red and the superficial capillary plexus (SCP) segmentation outlined in yellow.

OCTA outputs include the *en face* C scan flow images segmented at various levels. Additionally, OCTA machines can also display structural B-scans with flow signal overlay. Flow signal is depicted as solid-color pixels superimposed atop the grey-scale structural B-scan (Fig. 1.2.7).

2.1 | OCT Interpretation

OCT interpretation can be both qualitative and quantitative. At present, in order to fully evaluate an OCT image, both are important.

Qualitative Interpretation

In qualitative interpretation, the clinician reviews individual line scans (B-scans) imaging the areas of interest in the retina and makes a qualitative assessment of the presence, absence, or change from prior scans of pathology based on a knowledge of normal anatomy. B-scans can be rendered in a color-coded image or in a gray-scale image representing the reflectivity of the various layers. By comparing line scans performed over time, the course of the underlying disease and its response to treatment can be assessed.

When performing qualitative interpretation, it is important to be aware of the following issues:

▶ **Registration**: future line scans must be registered to past scans. In other words, the examiner must be certain that the precise anatomic area of interest is scanned similarly in future tests. All commercially available machines have the capability of registering future line scans to past scans.

▶ **Sampling error**: if only one or several line scans are examined, the true pathology may be missed. When doing qualitative interpretation, it is important that multiple line scans through the macula are examined.

▶ **Subjective evaluation**: by its nature, the lack of accurate quantitative numbers means that line scan interpretation will be individualized. In addition, it is hard to gauge the effects of pathology that is improving in one area of the macula but getting worse in another.

Zones of line scans can be qualitatively described as hyper-reflective or hyporeflective, and demonstrate shadowing or reverse shadowing. **Hyper-reflective** areas reflect more light than normal for a given region. On the gray-scale image, they appear whiter than the surrounding areas. Examples include epiretinal membranes and hard exudates. **Hyporeflective** areas reflect less light than the surrounding areas. Areas with a higher fluid content, e.g., intraretinal cysts, are usually hyporeflective. **Shadowing** occurs when there is increased absorption of light compared with the surrounding tissue. This causes optical shadowing and decreased visualization of the outer tissues. Vitreous debris, larger retinal vessels, hard exudates, and highly pigmented areas cause shadowing. **Reverse shadowing** occurs when there is loss/atrophy of pigmented tissue that allows excessive light to be transmitted through to the outer layers. The retinal pigment epithelium (RPE) is a major source of light absorption on OCT scanning, therefore atrophy of the RPE can cause reverse shadowing.

Qualitative interpretation of optical coherence tomography angiography (OCTA) images involves review of both the line scan and *en face* images of the different vascular slabs. *En face* OCTA images primarily reveal areas of flow versus non-flow. Examples of flow include the normal vasculature but also neovascularization. Patches of true flow loss where vasculature is normally expected suggest ischemic damage or, in the choriocapillaris, infiltrative disease. However, optical shadowing and areas of flow slower than the threshold for detection can also lead to areas of signal loss that appear as areas of non-flow.

Quantitative Interpretation

Quantitative interpretation of OCT scans relies on the ability of the OCT software to distinguish the inner and outer margins of the retina or sublayers (e.g., nerve fiber layer), referred to as segmentation, and accurately calculate retinal thickness and/or volume. Retinal thickness can then be compared with age-matched controls for assessment of normalcy and monitored over time to judge the progression or regression of disease. Subsequent scans can be registered by the OCT software so that measurements of retinal thickness are compared over the same area of the macula every time. These are usually presented as Early Treatment of Diabetic Retinopathy Study (ETDRS) grids or color-coded maps of retinal thickness. Proper segmentation is also important to the interpretation of OCTA images to assess the individual vascular plexi accurately. However, to date, metrics to quantify flow information have only been proposed by investigative studies and are not in clinical use.

When comparing quantitative OCT scans, it is important to compare scans obtained on the same machine, since different OCT machines draw the outer retinal boundary at different levels (ellipsoid zone [EZ], outer segment tips, RPE) and therefore may obtain different retinal thickness measurements on the same patient at the same visit.

The major drawback to quantitative assessment is that even in modern OCT machines, quantitative scans are prone to artifacts. For example, the machine software may inaccurately identify the inner or outer retinal boundaries, and the thickness measurement is therefore inaccurate. This is called software breakdown. Artifacts can induce errors in measurement making quantitative data inaccurate.

3.1 Artifacts on SD-OCT and OCTA

Artifacts can occur during image acquisition or analysis as a result of software, patient, or operator factors. It is important to identify artifacts because they may affect the qualitative or quantitative interpretation of images. This chapter will discuss artifacts that occur with spectral domain (SD)-OCT and OCT angiography (OCTA) scanning.

OCT Artifacts

Mirror Artifact

▸ Cause: This artifact occurs when the eye is positioned incorrectly or when the retinal features of interest span a large depth range (e.g., in scanning bullous detached retina). The OCT image is generated by interference between the sample beam and a reference beam. The sample beam is delayed in its return with respect to the reference beam and the reference beam therefore determines a zero delay line. The SD-OCT cannot distinguish between positive and negative delays and if the zero delay line is pushed so that it is at the surface of or beyond the surface of the retina, light from the retina may actually return sooner than the reference beam generating negative interference, which then generates an inverted OCT scan. Thus, as the OCT scanner is positioned closer to the retina, parts of the retina that are beyond the zero delay line appear folded. As the scanner is pushed even further, the entire retinal image may appear inverted and this is called the mirror artifact.

An interesting corollary to this is that whereas in some machines, such as the Zeiss Cirrus system, there is decreased resolution with the mirroring, in other machines this may be done deliberately to allow better interference of the reference beam with light reflected from the choroid and thus allow better visualization of the choroidal structures, something that most commercially available machines now exploit in Enhanced Depth Imaging protocols.

▸ Identification: Inverted, partly inverted, possibly poor resolution image.
▸ Correction: Patients will need to be re-scanned to correct this error (Fig. 3.1.1).

Vignetting

▸ Cause: This occurs when part of the OCT beam is blocked by the iris.
▸ Identification: This is typically characterized by a loss of signal over one side of the image.
▸ Correction: This can be corrected by repositioning the OCT machine so that it is the correct distance from the eye, and by observing the rendered fundus image so that there is no shadowing seen when acquiring the OCT image (Fig. 3.1.2).

Misalignment

▸ Cause: A misalignment artifact occurs when the ETDRS (Early Treatment Diabetic Retinopathy Study) grid in a quantitative volumetric scan is not centered on the fovea. This typically happens in patients with poor or eccentric fixation or poor attention.

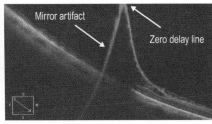
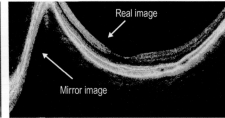
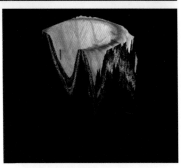

Figure 3.1.1 Shows mirror artifact in retinoschisis. The scanner is focused on the vitreoretinal surface at the site of the attached retina and the anteriorly projecting retinoschisis crosses the zero delay line giving a mirror image. The arrows point at the ghost image and the position of the zero delay line. The second image shows mirroring in a highly myopic eye with a long axial length. 3D reconstruction shows increased axial elongation of the highly myopic eye.

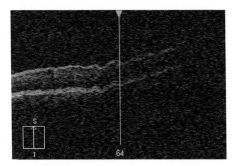

Figure 3.1.2 Peripheral vignetting is seen in a patient with a poorly dilated pupil. Note the poor image quality.

▸ Identification: In this situation, the normal foveal depression that usually appears blue on the ETDRS map is not aligned with the center of the ETDRS macular grid.
▸ Correction: We can manually correct misalignment on most SD-OCT machines. Alternatively, the patient can be rescanned using external fixation (Fig. 3.1.3).

Software Breakdown

▸ Cause: OCT segmentation lines to calculate retinal thickness and topographic maps are automatically drawn by the OCT machine. The inner line is drawn at the internal limiting membrane (ILM) and the outer line is drawn either at the level of the RPE (Cirrus, Optvue) or at the inner segment–outer segment (IS-OS) junction or photoreceptor OS tips. Software breakdown can cause misidentification of either the inner or outer

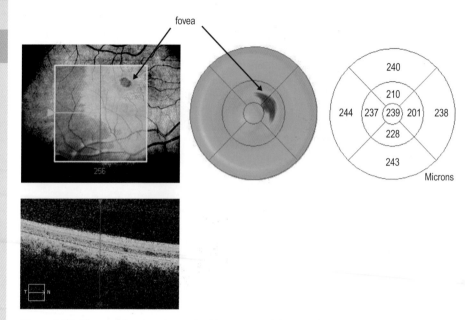

fovea

256

240

210

244 237 239 201 238

228

243

Microns

Figure 3.1.3 The macular map shows the thinnest part of the macula eccentric to the center of the Early Treatment Diabetic Retinopathy Study grid and the rendered fundus image. Note the absence of the foveal pit in the center of the line scan.

retinal boundary. This happens most commonly because of poor-quality scans, retinal pathology, or the presence of media opacity. This results in inaccurate mapping and quantitative measurements.

Generally, SD-OCT is better than time domain (TD)-OCT in avoiding these misalignment errors.

Inner-line breakdown typically happens in vitreomacular surface disorders such as vitreomacular traction (VMT) or epiretinal membrane formation. Because macular thickness maps are less likely to be used for critical therapeutic decision-making in these situations, this type of software breakdown is less significant. Outer-line breakdown happens in conditions involving the outer retina/retinal pigment epithelium (RPE) such as central serous chorioretinopathy (CSCR), age-related macular degeneration (AMD), cystoid macular edema (CME), and retinal atrophy. In some cases, such as CSCR, these errors may be critically important if retinal thickness maps drive therapeutic decisions.

▶ Identification: Software breakdown should be suspected when the macular map has a "bowtie" appearance or when there are isolated islands of retinal thinning or thickening on the OCT map that are inconsistent with the clinical picture.
▶ Correction: Some OCT machines allow manual correction of segmentation errors to obtain more accurate thickness readings. Alternatively, the patient can be rescanned (Figs. 3.1.4 and 3.1.5).

Blink Artifact

▶ Cause: This happens when a patient blinks during OCT image acquisition. The scanning beam is blocked momentarily and this results in a black bar on the OCT image and the macular map.

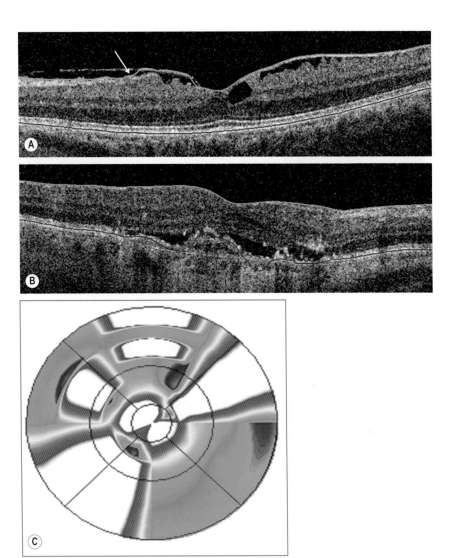

Figure 3.1.4 Shows inner (A) and outer (B) line software breakdown. (C) Shows the "bowtie" appearance of the macular map with inner line breakdown.

▶ Identification: The blink artifact can be identified by an obvious area of dropout on an individual B-scan, a black or white bar across the *en face* image, or obviously incorrect thinning shown on the macular thickness map.

▶ Correction: If clinically necessary, the scan can be redone. Artificial tears may be used to lubricate the eyes prior to scanning (Fig. 3.1.6).

Motion Artifact

▶ Cause: This occurs when there is movement of the eye during OCT scanning leading to distortion or double scanning of the same area. Motion can be axial or transverse and can occur because of poor fixation tracking of the light source, heartbeat, respiration, drifts, or saccades. It can cause errors especially in quantitative measurements.

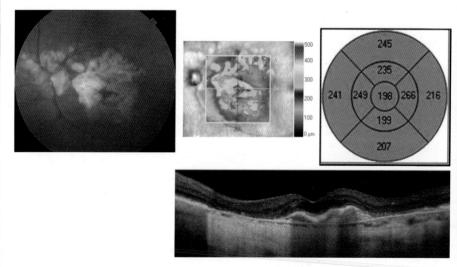

Figure 3.1.5 Shows outer-line breakdown in an eye with macular geographic atrophy.

▸ Identification: Motion is seen on B scans as a sharp change in contour or blurring and on the *en face* image as misalignment of blood vessels. Improved speed in SD-OCT reduces drift and motion artifacts but may manifest a double fovea artifact with motion.

▸ Correction: This artifact can be corrected by redoing the scan, trying a faster scanning protocol, or using a tracking system where available on the commercial OCT machines (Fig. 3.1.6)

Out of Range Error

▸ Cause: This is an operator-induced error where a section of the OCT scan is cut off because the B-scan is vertically shifted out of the scanning range.

▸ Identification: Cut-off of the top (inner retinal) or bottom (choroidal) part of the OCT scan.

▸ Correction: This can only be corrected by rescanning (Fig. 3.1.7).

OCTA Artifacts

OCTA is an extension of OCT. As such, some artifacts mentioned in the previous section are also seen on OCTA scans. Other artifacts are unique to OCTA's flow detection capacity and will be detailed in this section.

Motion Artifact

▸ Cause: Like motion artifact on OCT, this artifact occurs when there is motion of the eye during OCTA scanning.

▸ Identification: On B-scans with flow overlay, motion is seen as blurring of the retinal layers and confluent flow pixels. On the *en face* image, motion will appear as horizontal lines at locations where OCTA data were not collected and will be seen as discontinuity, blurring, or duplication of vessels. This artifact can cause errors in quantitative metrics such as vessel density and FAZ area.

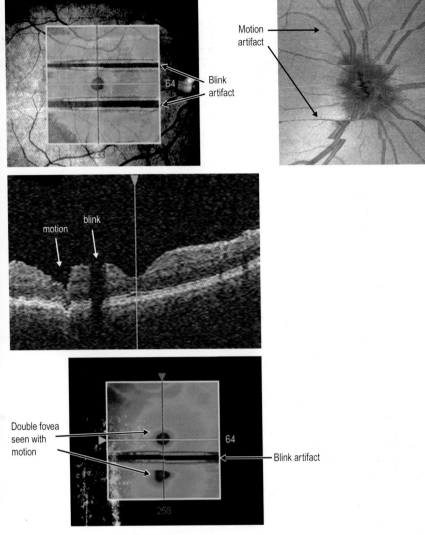

Figure 3.1.6 Blink artifact is seen as a dark line across the image. Motion artifact is seen as the discontinuity of the retinal vasculature in the first two rendered fundus images. The third image shows a double fovea exclusive to SD-OCT where rapid scanning of the eye captures the fovea twice as it moves.

▶ Correction: This artifact can be corrected with the use of eye-tracking and software motion correction available on many OCTA devices. If these technologies are not available, rescanning or selecting a shorter scan pattern will often correct the artifact (Fig. 3.1.8).

Shadowing

▶ Cause: Shadowing occurs when the OCTA beam cannot reach the outer retinal layers. It is caused by blockage of the beam by pathologic features such as hemorrhage, vitreous floaters, and drusen. Pathologic features are often reflective and prohibit the OCTA beam from properly assessing underlying areas. As a result, areas below these features will appear as flow-voids on *en face* angiography.

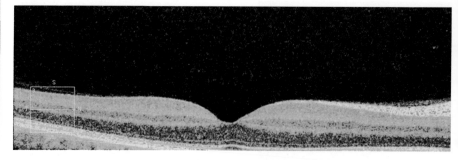

Figure 3.1.7 The choroidal side of the image is cut off because of improper positioning.

▸ Identification: Proper identification of shadowing artifact requires assessing the structural *en face* image and angiogram together. The structural *en face* image will show reduced signal in areas where the OCT beam has been blocked. Areas with low signal on the structural *en face* or structural B-scan image are prone to shadowing artifact and should not be interpreted as true flow voids on angiography.

▸ Correction: In the case of mobile sources of shadowing, such as vitreous floaters, rescanning can correct the artifact. For other causes of shadowing, such as hemorrhage and drusen, little can be done for immediate correction. Although the longer wavelength of swept-source devices allows slightly improved penetration, shadowing is still an issue in these devices (Fig. 3.1.9).

Projection Artifact

▸ Cause: Projection artifact occurs when the OCTA beam reaches the RPE, a natural reflector. As the beam passes through the inner retina, it is distorted by flow in the superficial capillary plexus. When the beam is reflected off the RPE, the distorted light is misinterpreted as a decorrelation signal in the outer retinal layers. This creates the appearance of flow in the outer retinal layers that mirrors that of the superficial capillary plexus and/or large retinal vessels.

▸ Identification: Nearly all OCTA scans contain projection artifacts. *En face* images of the outer retinal layers will show large vessels belonging to the superficial capillary plexus. This artifact is easily identified on B-scans, where projection artifacts appear as flow tails (e.g., decorrelation tails) trailing below superficial vessels.

▸ Correction: Most OCTA devices offer projection artifact removal. Correction is based on removing the decorrelation signal of superficial vascular layers from underlying angiograms (Fig. 3.1.10).

Segmentation Artifact

▸ Cause: Segmentation artifacts occur when OCTA software cannot properly identify retinal layer boundaries. It is caused by pathology, such as fluid and drusen, that distorts normal retinal anatomy. It can lead to improper selection of retinal slabs and erroneous vessel quantification and pathology identification.

▸ Identification: B-scans will show segmentation boundaries at anatomically incorrect locations.

▸ Correction: OCTA devices offer manual segmentation to correct this error. However, manual segmentation is time consuming and not adaptable to clinical practice. Adjusting segmentation along the z-axis can serve as a method for coarse correction when clinically necessary (Fig. 3.1.11).

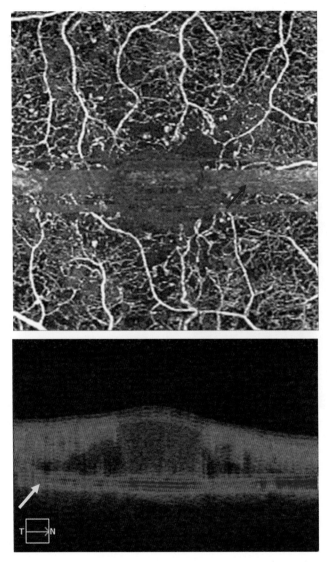

Figure 3.1.8 Motion artifact is seen as a horizontal line across the *en face* image (red arrow). The second image shows blurred boundaries and spurious flow detection on a B-scan (yellow arrow).

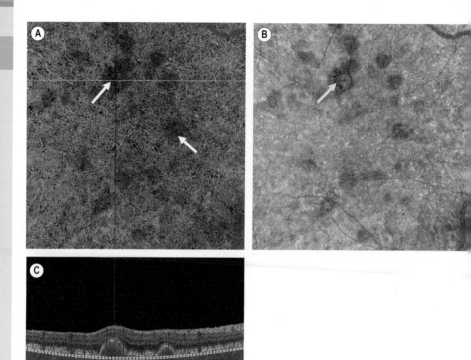

Figure 3.1.9 Shadowing effect of drusen on the choriocapillaris of a patient with intermediate AMD. (A) An OCTA at the level of the choriocapillaris showing dark areas (white arrows) that could reflect either flow voids or shadowing. (B) An intensity/structural *en face* image showing signal reduction under the drusen thereby confirming that the dark area in (A) is shadowing and not a flow void (yellow arrow). (C) A B-scan through the drusen showing shadowing under the drusen (white arrowheads).

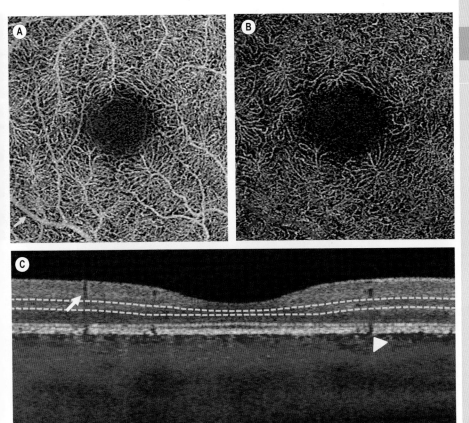

Figure 3.1.10 (A) *En face* image of the deep capillary plexus without projection artifact removal shows overlying superficial retinal vessels (yellow arrow). (B) shows the same image after software correction for projection artifact. Note that the software has removed large projected superficial vessels (red arrow). (C) The cross-sectional B-scan for parts (A) and (B). The white arrow points to a decorrelation tail arising from a superficial retinal vessel and the arrowhead points to the reflection of an overlying vessel at the level of the retinal pigment epithelium.

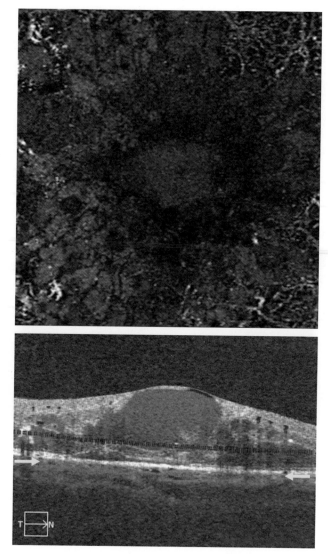

Figure 3.1.11 *En face* image of the choriocapillaris slab in a patient with diabetic macular edema. The second image shows the B-scan with misidentified segmentation boundaries caused by macular edema. The yellow arrows point to the boundaries' correct location.

4.1 | Normal Retinal Anatomy and Basic Pathologic Appearances

Normal Retinal Anatomy

Commercially available spectral domain (SD-OCT) scanners have an Axial Resolution of between 4 μm and 7 μm and a transverse resolution of approximately 15 μm. Swept source (SS-OCT) devices, on the other hand, have an axial resolution between 6.3 μm and 8 μm and a transverse resolution of 20 μm. This high resolution allows for exquisite viewing of the retinal detail. Due to the limited penetration of light beyond the pigmented retinal pigment epithelium (RPE) and the drop-off of the OCT signal with depth (also called sensitivity roll-off), the image at the level of the choroid has a lower resolution. Swept source technology provides less sensitivity roll off and therefore can image the choroid better than SD-OCT. The layers of the normal retina are labeled in Figure 4.1.1.

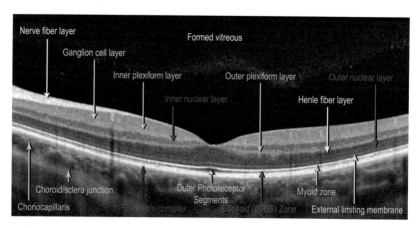

Figure 4.1.1 Normal retinal anatomy.

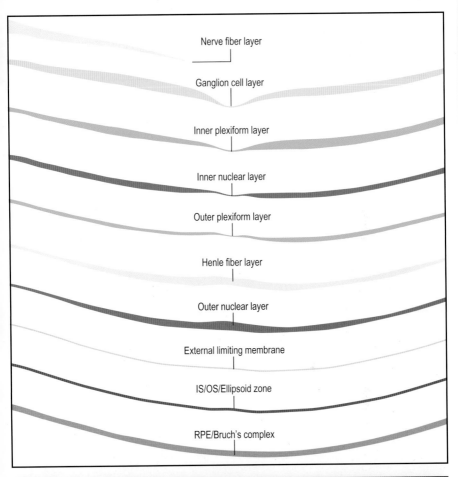

Nerve fiber layer

Ganglion cell layer

Inner plexiform layer

Inner nuclear layer

Outer plexiform layer

Henle fiber layer

Outer nuclear layer

External limiting membrane

IS/OS/Ellipsoid zone

RPE/Bruch's complex

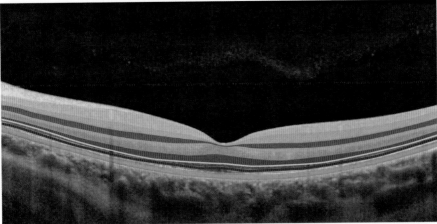

Figure 4.1.1 *Continued.*

Additional Vitreous Features

Some additional vitreous features are demonstrated in a normal OCT scan in Figure 4.1.2:

▸ Posterior cortical vitreous (posterior hyaloid)
▸ Retro-hyaloidal space

Normal Vasculature

OCT angiography (OCTA) helps visualize the distinct layers of capillary beds in the retina. The superficial capillary plexus and deep capillary plexus are derived from the retinal circulation and nourish the inner two-thirds of the retina while the choriocapillaris is part of the choroidal circulation and helps supply the outer retina (Fig. 4.1.3).

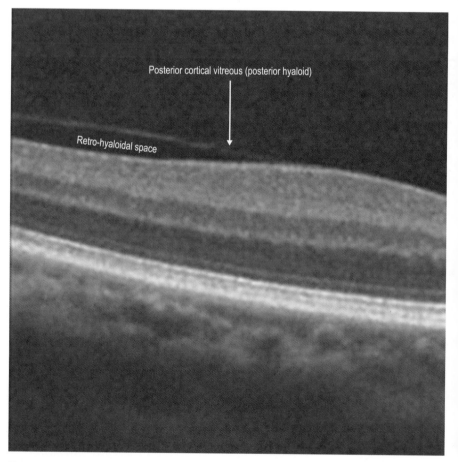

Figure 4.1.2 Vitreous features in a normal eye with partial, shallow vitreous separation.

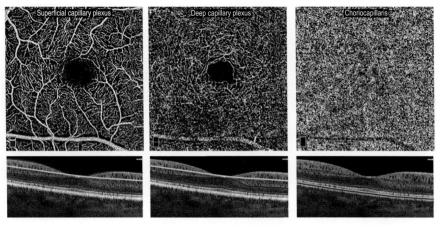

Figure 4.1.3 *En face* OCTA images of the superficial capillary plexus, deep capillary plexus, and choriocapillaris in a normal eye with corresponding B-scan through the fovea showing the segmentation lines.

General Appearance of Retinal Pathology on SD-OCT

Cystic Changes in Outer Retina

Discrete hyporeflective spaces are noticed primarily in the outer retina, but usually span multiple layers (Fig. 4.1.4).

The differential diagnosis includes:
▸ Diabetic macular edema
▸ Branch retinal vein obstruction
▸ Central retinal vein obstruction
▸ Retinal telangiectasias (e.g., Coat's disease, macular telangiectasia)
▸ Retinitis pigmentosa
▸ Uveitis/retinal vasculitis
▸ Post surgery
▸ Nicotinic acid maculopathy
▸ Vitreomacular disorders (vitreomacular traction, epiretinal membrane)
▸ Chronic subretinal fluid (e.g., retinal detachment, choroidal neovascular membrane, central serous chorioretinopathy)
▸ Idiopathic

Subretinal Fluid

Clear hyporeflective space can be seen between the neurosensory retina and the RPE (Fig. 4.1.5).

The differential diagnosis includes:
▸ Central serous chorioretinopathy
▸ Choroidal neovascular membranes (secondary to, e.g., age-related macular degeneration, myopia)
▸ Serous retinal detachments (secondary to tumors, inflammation, trauma)
▸ Rhegmatogenous retinal detachment
▸ Tractional retinal detachment

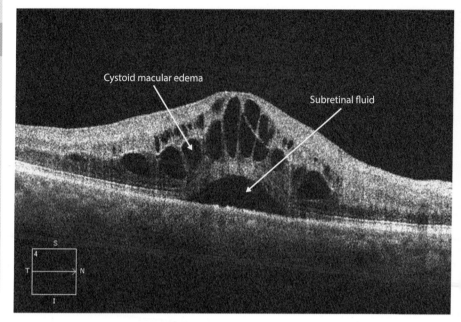

Figure 4.1.4 Cystoid changes in retina.

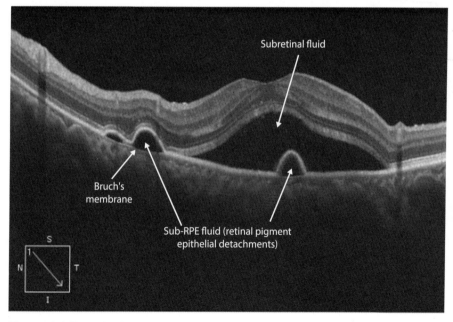

Figure 4.1.5 Clear subretinal fluid.

TURBID SUBRETINAL FLUID

Subretinal fluid may be turbid or have a higher reflectivity than the vitreous in conditions where there is fibrin deposition in the subretinal space (Fig. 4.1.6).

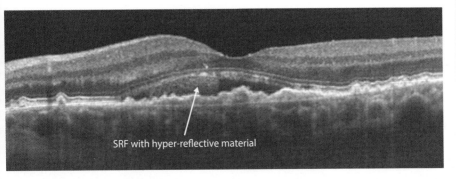

SRF with hyper-reflective material

Figure 4.1.6 Turbid subretinal fluid (SRF).

▸ The differential diagnosis includes
▸ Chronic central serous chorioretinopathy
▸ Chronic choroidal neovascular membrane
▸ Sympathetic ophthalmia
▸ Vogt–Koyanagi–Harada syndrome
▸ Inflammatory serous retinal detachments.

Retinal Pigment Epithelial Detachment

This is noted as a dome-shaped separation of the RPE from the underlying Bruch's membrane. The ensuing space between the RPE and Bruch's membrane is hyporeflective (Fig. 4.1.7). A low-lying, irregular pigment epithelial detachment is called a double layer sign, which refers to the visibility of both the RPE and Bruch's membrane as separate layers on OCT with hyporeflective space in between (Fig. 4.1.6), and is often indicative of a choroidal neovascularization.

The differential diagnosis includes:
▸ Age-related macular degeneration
▸ Central serous chorioretinopathy
▸ Choroidal neovascularization (e.g., myopic degeneration, presumed ocular histoplasmosis, angioid streaks)
▸ Idiopathic

RPE Atrophy

Atrophy of the pigmented RPE causes decreased absorption of light. The OCT signal is therefore able to penetrate more deeply, which exaggerates the typical signal pattern so that there is a reverse shadowing effect (Fig. 4.1.8, area between the smaller arrows).

The differential diagnosis includes:
▸ Geographic atrophy secondary to age-related macular degeneration
▸ Advanced chorioretinal scarring secondary to retinal degenerations and macular dystrophies (e.g., retinitis pigmentosa, Stargardt's disease, cone dystrophy)
▸ Chorioretinal atrophy secondary to inflammatory disorders (e.g., ocular histoplasmosis, multifocal choroiditis)
▸ Severe myopic degeneration
▸ Angioid streaks

Normal Retinal Anatomy and Basic Pathologic Appearances

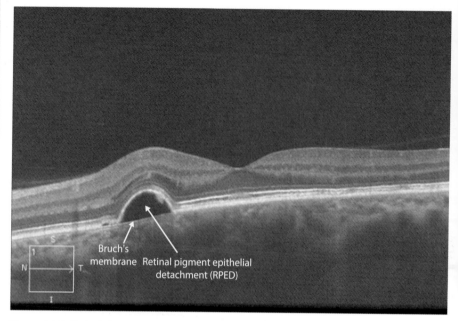

Figure 4.1.7 Retinal pigment epithelial detachment.

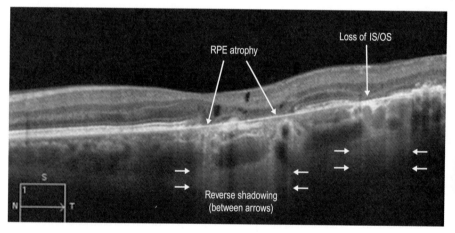

Figure 4.1.8 RPE atrophy and loss of photoreceptors with mild cystic change in the retina.

Focal Loss of External Limiting Membrane (ELM) and Inner Segment–Outer Segment (IS–OS) Photoreceptor Junction

OCT scanning reveals a disruption in the ELM line and in the ellipsoid zone (also referred to as the IS–OS/photoreceptor junction) (Fig. 4.1.9). Loss of the IS–OS junction and ELM has been associated with reduction in visual acuity and a worse prognosis for visual recovery in a number of ocular disorders. Some diseases can present with outer retinal disruption in the early stages, but almost all degenerative conditions of the retinal can show outer retinal loss with sufficiently advanced disease.

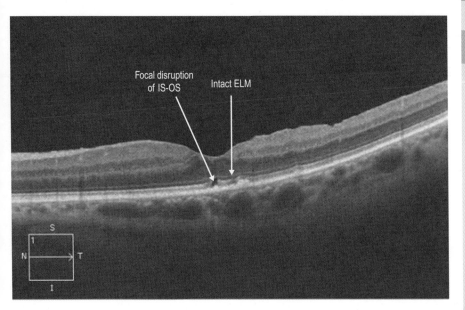

Figure 4.1.9 Focal loss of the IS-OS junction.

The differential diagnosis includes:
- Cone dystrophy
- End-stage rod dystrophy
- Solar retinopathy
- Syphilis
- Inflammatory disease (e.g., multiple evanescent white dot syndrome, acute posterior multifocal placoid pigment epitheliopathy)
- Degenerative disorders of the outer retina such as age-related macular degeneration
- Disorders associated with long-standing macular edema, which can eventually cause outer retinal atrophy

Vitreous Opacities

Posterior vitreous opacities are seen as hyper-reflective specks in the vitreous space (Fig. 4.1.10).

The differential diagnosis includes:
- Vitritis
- Asteroid hyalosis
- Syneresis scintillans
- Operculum (e.g., related to a macular hole)
- Fungal hyphae

General Appearance of Vascular Pathology on OCTA

Choroidal or Macular Neovascularization (MNV)

Macular neovascularization (MNV) often appears as an irregular network of vessels at the level of the outer (generally avascular) retina or under the retinal pigment epithelium (Fig. 4.1.11). Type 1 MNV is typically best visualized in the choriocapillaris slab, and type 2 neovascularization will yield flow signal in the otherwise avascular outer retinal slab. Type 3 neovascularization can be hard to visualize *en face*, but the OCT B-scan will

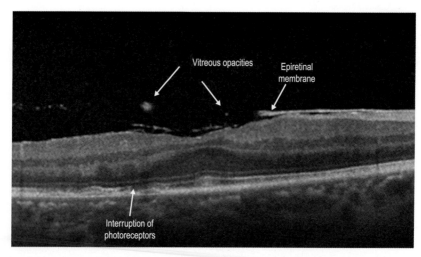

Figure 4.1.10 Vitreous opacities.

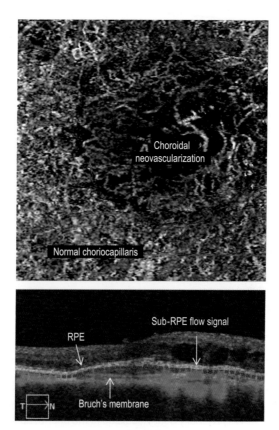

Figure 4.1.11 Neovascular vessels in the choriocapillaris slab on OCTA and the corresponding flow overlay and segmentation lines atop the structural B-scan.

show flow pixels in the avascular outer retina and may show these extending beneath the RPE.

The differential diagnosis includes:
- Wet age-related macular degeneration
- Pathologic myopia
- Angioid streaks
- Ocular histoplasmosis
- Central serous chorioretinopathy

Retinal Neovascularization

Neovascularization of the retinal vessels, such as in proliferative diabetic retinopathy, is best visualized *en face* in the vitreomacular interface (VMI) slab.

The differential diagnosis includes:
- Proliferative diabetic retinopathy
- Other retinal ischemic diseases (e.g., sickle cell disease, retinal vein obstruction)

Capillary Dropout

Dark areas in the retinal capillary plexi where flow signal is otherwise expected are referred to as capillary dropout or capillary non-perfusion, which is typically indicative of ischemia and resultant loss of flow in the capillaries (Fig. 4.1.12).

The differential diagnosis includes:
- Diabetic retinopathy
- Branch or central retinal vein obstruction
- Branch or central retinal artery obstruction

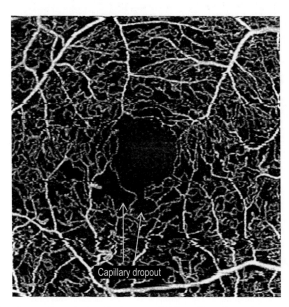

Capillary dropout

Figure 4.1.12 Macular capillary dropout in the superficial capillary plexus from a patient with diabetic retinopathy.

Flow Deficit

This term is similar to capillary dropout but refers to loss of flow signal in the choriocapillaris. Beyond ischemic damage, loss of flow signal can also be attributed to compression of the choriocapillaris. When evaluating for a choriocapillaris flow deficit, it is important to differentiate it from shadowing of overlying structures, which may also appear dark like a flow deficit. Differentiation is made by looking for shadowing on the corresponding B-scans and for loss of signal on the corresponding *en face* intensity image (Fig. 4.1.13).

The differential diagnosis of choriocapillaris flow deficits includes:

▸ Choroiditis (e.g., acute posterior multifocal placoid pigment epitheliopathy, birdshot chorioretinopathy)
▸ Sarcoidosis
▸ Choroidal tumors
▸ Central serous choroidopathy
▸ Geographic atrophy
▸ Normal aging

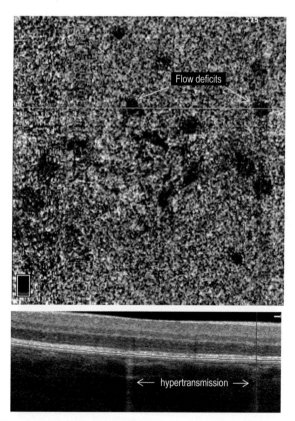

Figure 4.1.13 Flow deficits in the choriocapillaris. The green line corresponds to the location of the B-scan, which runs through two flow deficits. Hyper-transmission on the B-scan shows the dark areas are truly choriocapillaris dropout and not just shadowing.

Microaneurysms

These are seen as focal areas of dilated capillary segments or capillary loops (Fig. 4.1.14).
The differential diagnosis includes:
▹ Diabetic retinopathy
▹ Ocular ischemic syndrome

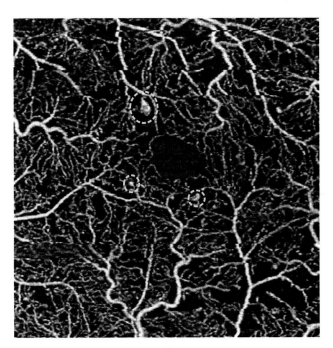

Figure 4.1.14 Microaneurysms in the superficial capillary plexus.

PART 2: Optic Nerve Disorders

Section 5: Optic Nerve Disorders...38

    5.1   *Basic Optic Nerve Scan Patterns and Output* 38
           Daniela Ferrara, Alexandre S.C. Reis, and Alessandro A. Jammal

5.1 | Basic Optic Nerve Scan Patterns and Output

Commercially available SD-OCT machines have three basic scan patterns used to evaluate the optic nerve head (ONH), the peripapillary retinal nerve fiber layer (RNFL), and the macular area:

▸ Volume scans: these are analogous to macular cube scans in which a volumetric set of data centered on the ONH is acquired. These may be square or rectangular cubes of data around the optic nerve. The Cirrus HD-OCT scanning protocol generates a cube of data through a 6-mm square grid by acquiring a series of 200 horizontal B-scans, each composed of 200 A-scans (Fig. 5.1.1). In addition, the scan pattern overlays concentric rings to assist in the alignment of the optic disc. Software processing within the device then identifies the center of the optic disc and creates a 3.46-mm circle centered on this location for registration purposes. The data set is then used to measure peripapillary RNFL thickness. The RTVue ONH scan pattern consists of a grid pattern with circular and radial scans that acquires a 4 mm × 4 mm volume around the ONH (Fig. 5.1.1). The machines also have the ability to acquire cubes of data centered on the fovea to measure the ganglion cell complex (GCC) layers as part of the glaucoma imaging protocol. Most of them do macula and optic disc scans separately, but the Topcon Triton acquires a 3D wide scan of 12 mm × 9 mm (512 × 256 pixels), which allows simultaneous ONH, peripapillary RNFL, and macular analysis (Fig. 5.1.1).

▸ Circle scans: The Heidelberg Spectralis SD-OCT glaucoma protocol acquires a set of three sequential and concentric peripapillary circular scans centered on the ONH, each with 768 A-scans subtending 12, 14, and 16 degrees (3.5 mm, 4.1 mm, and 4.7 mm in diameter, respectively) to measure peripapillary RNFL thickness (Fig. 5.1.1).

▸ Line scans: a single or a series of high-resolution B-scans can be obtained across the ONH, similar to the line scans obtained in the macula, to allow higher-resolution visualization of structures and anatomic anomalies of the ONH. Line scans are also used as radial patterns, centered on the optic disc allowing the acquisition of additional parameters (i.e., minimum rim width).

The information obtained from the ONH volumetric scans is processed to obtain the following parameters:

Retinal Nerve Fiber Layer Thickness

The RNFL thickness is calculated as the distance between the internal limiting membrane and the outer boundary of the RNFL (Fig. 5.1.2). Most machines calculate the RNFL thickness along a circle of a predefined diameter (usually between 3.4 and 3.5 mm) centered on the optic disc (Fig. 5.1.1). One of the reasons that measurement of the RNFL between machines is not comparable is that different machines use circles of different diameters. RNFL thickness is then compared with age, ethnicity, and disc size-matched normative databases. The results are displayed in various forms including a false color scale where green represents normal, yellow represents a borderline RNFL thickness (less than 5% and greater than 1% probability of being normal), and red represents an abnormal RNFL thickness (less than 1% probability of being normal). Results from the two eyes are also compared and any discrepancy between the two is highlighted. The RNFL thickness may be displayed as an average for the overall map, quadrants, sectors, hemispheres, and/or clock hours.

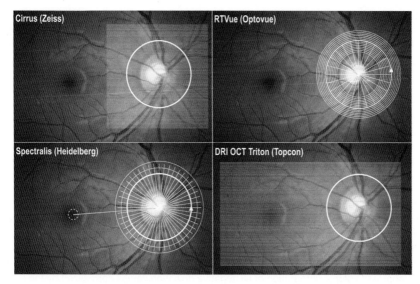

Figure 5.1.1 Composite showing the optic nerve head and peripapillary area scan patterns used for each device.

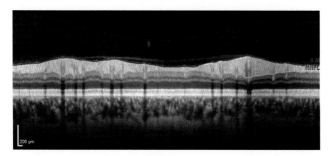

Figure 5.1.2 Circle B-scan of the peripapillary retina. Assessment of the retinal nerve fiber layer (RNFL) thickness with OCT requires accurate delineation of the limits of the RNFL by the instrument's software. The red line represents the internal limiting membrane and the turquoise line the outer limits of the RNFL. These boundaries are found by a threshold procedure, in which differences in reflectance between outer and inner retinal structures are interpreted as different layers.

One of the most useful RNFL displays in clinical practice is the sinusoidal profile wave corresponding to the RNFL thickness profile 360 degrees around the optic nerve, starting from the temporal region and proceeding through the superior, nasal, inferior, and back to the temporal region (TSNIT). The RNFL thickness profile normally presents a 'double hump' pattern corresponding to the superior and inferior quadrants, where the RNFL is thicker.

Optic Nerve Morphology

The software in various SD-OCT machines also calculates and displays the optic disc area, cup and rim areas, volumes for cup and rim, cup-to-disc ratios, and cup-to-disc horizontal and vertical ratios. The Heidelberg Spectralis SD-OCT uses 24 high-resolution radially equidistant B-scans. Internal software provides automatic segmentations of the internal limiting membrane and for the 48 Bruch's membrane opening points (one on each side of the

B-scan). The minimum rim width is defined as the minimum distance between the Bruch's membrane opening and the internal limiting membrane; it is calculated independently for each of the 24 radial B-scans (48 measurements per eye) and averaged for a global value.

Ganglion Cell Complex (GCC)

The GCC consists of three inner retinal layers: the RNFL (axons of the ganglion cells), the ganglion cell layer (cell bodies of the ganglion cells), and the inner plexiform layer (dendrites of the ganglion cells). The GCC scan is a series of B-scans centered on the macula to quantify the thickness in all of these three layers. After image processing, GCC thickness is calculated as the distance between the internal limiting membrane and the outer boundary of the inner plexiform layer. Some machines use the ganglion cell layer in isolation or a combination of the three layers. The software presents the results as a color-coded map that compares the examined eye with a normative database and indicates deviations from normal values. The GCC scan must be centered precisely on the fovea to have its results compared with a normative database or to permit progression analysis.

The GCC thickness analysis may be displayed as an average overall thickness, averages in the superior and inferior hemiretina, superior–inferior difference in GCC thickness, the global loss volume (integration of all negative deviation values normalized by the overall map area), and the focal loss volume (integration of negative deviation values in the areas of significant focal loss).

PART 3: Macular Disorders

Section 6: **Dry Age-Related Macular Degeneration** 42
  6.1   Dry Age-Related Macular Degeneration 42

Section 7: **Wet Age-Related Macular Degeneration** 46
  7.1   Wet Age-Related Macular Degeneration 46

Section 8: **Macular Pathology Associated With Myopia** 56
  8.1   Posterior Staphyloma 56
  8.2   Myopic Choroidal Neovascular Membrane 58
  8.3   Myopic Macular Schisis 62
  8.4   Dome-Shaped Macula 64
  8.5   Myopic Tractional Retinal Detachment 66

Section 9: **Vitreomacular Interface Disorders** 68
  9.1   Pachychoroid Syndromes 68
        Luísa S.M. Mendonça
  9.2   Vitreomacular Adhesion and Vitreomacular Traction 74
        Omar Abu-Qamar
  9.3   Full-Thickness Macular Hole 78
        Emily S. Levine
  9.4   Lamellar Macular Hole 82
        Emily S. Levine
  9.5   Epiretinal Membrane 84
        Emily S. Levine

Section 10: **Miscellaneous Causes of Macular Edema** 88
  10.1 Postoperative Cystoid Macular Edema 88
  10.2 Macular Telangiectasia 90
  10.3 Uveitis 96

Section 11: **Miscellaneous Macular Disorders** 100
  11.1 Central Serous Chorioretinopathy 100
        Omar Abu-Qamar
  11.2 Hydroxychloroquine Toxicity 104
  11.3 Pattern Dystrophy 108
  11.4 Oculocutaneous Albinism 112
  11.5 Subretinal Perfluorocarbon 114
  11.6 X-Linked Juvenile Retinoschisis 116

Introduction: Dry age-related macular degeneration (AMD) accounts for a significant degree of visual disability in elderly populations. Loss of vision is secondary to photoreceptor cell death, which manifests clinically as geographic atrophy (GA). The dry form of AMD comprises approximately 85% of all AMD cases and currently has no available effective treatment.

Clinical Features: The hallmark feature of dry AMD is the presence of drusen, which are yellow-colored subretinal deposits that range in size and appearance (Fig. 6.1.1). Small, fine drusen without other manifestations such as retinal pigment epithelium (RPE) changes or atrophy should not be considered AMD. Additionally, there can be varied pigmentary changes within the RPE. Advanced forms of AMD feature atrophy of the RPE with eventual GA (Figs. 6.1.2 and 6.1.3), which can occur in the presence or absence of drusen.

OCT Features: **Drusen** are identified on OCT by their characteristic appearance as **discrete elevations of the RPE layer with medium reflectance** at the level of Bruch's membrane (Figs. 6.1.4 and 6.1.5). Drusen may be of varying size and contour. Drusen can be described histopathologically as **basal linear**, when the deposits occur between the basement membrane of the RPE and Bruch's membrane (more typical), or **basal laminar**, when the deposits occur between the plasma membrane of the RPE and the basement membrane of the RPE. Basal

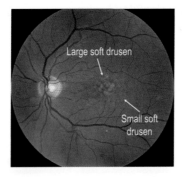

Figure 6.1.1 Color fundus photograph of dry AMD with many soft drusen of varying size.

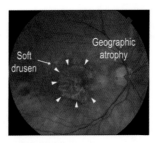

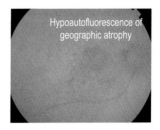

Figure 6.1.3 Fundus autofluorescence image (corresponding to Figure 6.1.1) highlights areas of geographic atrophy as distinct areas of hypoautofluorescence.

Figure 6.1.2 Color fundus photograph of a large area of central geographic atrophy (arrowheads) and surrounding soft drusen.

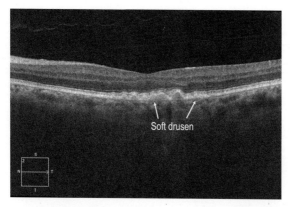

Figure 6.1.4 OCT (corresponding to Figure 6.1.1) showing features of dry AMD. There are many discrete, round, hill-shaped elevations below the RPE, which are basal linear drusen (arrows). Drusen exhibit a medium-intensity reflectance pattern on OCT.

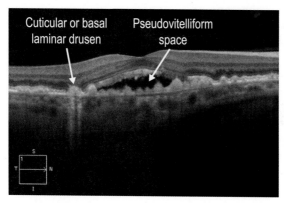

Figure 6.1.5 OCT showing basal laminar or cuticular drusen. An associated pseudo-vitelliform detachment is present in the macula, which can be seen in the setting of cuticular drusen, even in the absence of choroidal neovascularization.

laminar drusen are also called **cuticular** drusen and are characteristically small and regular shaped in a diffuse arrangement within the macula. It is difficult to distinguish between basal linear and basal laminar drusen on OCT. **GA** is identified by absence of the outer retinal layers and RPE, which leads to a **reverse shadowing effect** (Figs. 6.1.6 and 6.1.7). The choroidal thickness is typically less than normal in AMD.

Ancillary Testing: Color fundus photographs and fundus autofluorescence can be helpful to highlight and track areas of GA (Fig. 6.1.3).

Treatment: No treatment is currently available for dry AMD although numerous research endeavors are underway, particularly for the treatment of GA.

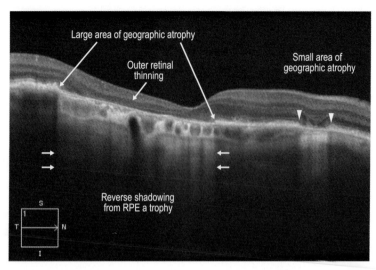

Figure 6.1.6 OCT (corresponding to Figure 6.1.2) showing larger (between arrows) and smaller (between arrowheads) areas of GA. In areas of GA, there is loss of the outer retinal layers and RPE. Due to absence of the RPE in these areas, the OCT signal is able to penetrate deeper, which exaggerates the typical signal pattern so that there is a reverse shadowing effect.

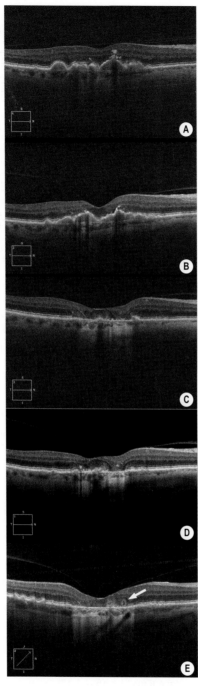

Figure 6.1.7 OCT natural progression of dry AMD over a 6-year period. Numerous, large drusenoid pigment epithelial detachments are present along with pigmentary migration within the retina at baseline (**A**), which coalesce and begin to flatten over time (**B**), with eventual progression to patchy geographic atrophy (**C**, **D**), followed by diffuse subfoveal geographic atrophy (**E**). Outer retinal tubulation and cysts over atrophy are common features of advanced dry AMD and may be mistaken for evidence of wet AMD (arrow).

Introduction: Wet (neovascular, exudative) age-related macular degeneration (AMD) is a leading cause of severe vision loss in the elderly population of developed societies. It represents approximately 10% of all AMD cases.

Clinical Features: The distinguishing feature is the presence of choroidal neovascularization (CNV) in the setting of a patient over the age of 60 years, virtually always with some manifestations of concurrent or preexisting dry AMD (drusen, geographic atrophy, retinal pigment epithelium [RPE] abnormalities). CNV results in leakage of fluid and/or hemorrhage within or underneath the neurosensory retina, and/or underneath the RPE and, if untreated, results in permanent photoreceptor damage and scarring. On the basis of fluorescein angiography, CNV can be subtyped into classic, occult, or mixed types. An OCT-based anatomic classification divides CNV into type 1 or occult (below the RPE), type 2 or classic (above the RPE), and type 3 or retinal angiomatosis proliferation [RAP] (intraretinal). Type 1 CNV are the most frequently encountered subtype, although mixed type CNV are frequently present. OCT angiography (OCTA) provides a more precise manner in separating out various CNV anatomical locales compared with other macular imaging modalities. In the presence of a large pigment epithelial detachment (PED), a tear of the RPE can occur. End-stage wet AMD may result in disciform scar formation.

OCT Features: The most characteristic findings on OCT in wet AMD are the presence of an **irregularly shaped PED** with adjacent **subretinal hemorrhage** and **subretinal fluid**. An irregularly shaped PED is in contrast to a more smooth-shaped PED typically seen in central serous chorioretinopathy. In wet AMD, especially in type 2 CNV, there is frequently a visible interruption in the RPE layer. The following are various key features of wet AMD that can be uniquely identified based on their OCT appearance:

▸ **Classic CNV:** a classic, or type 2, CNV is present when the abnormal neovascular tissue penetrates the RPE/Bruch's membrane complex and is present in the subretinal space (Figs. 7.1.1–7.1.4).
▸ **Occult CNV:** an occult, or type 1, CNV is present when the abnormal neovascular tissue remains underneath the RPE (Figs. 7.1.5–7.1.8).
▸ **RPE tear:** an RPE tear has a very characteristic OCT appearance (Figs. 7.1.9 and 7.1.10), where there is a sharply demarcated region of absent RPE adjacent to an area of bunched-up RPE.
▸ **Disciform scar:** a disciform scar can have a varied OCT appearance but is always dominated by a hyper-reflective subretinal scar (Figs. 7.1.11 and 7.1.12).
▸ **Treated CNV:** following treatment with anti-vascular endothelial growth factor (anti-VEGF) therapy, intra- and subretinal fluid will often improve significantly or completely resolve (Figs. 7.1.13 and 7.1.14). Associated PEDs also tend to decrease in size with continued treatment.
▸ **Retinal angiomatous proliferation:** type 3 neovascularization (or RAP) is a less common cause of exudative AMD resulting from abnormal neovascular tissue within the deep retina that typically originates within the retina and migrates towards the choriocapillaris and/or retinal surface (Figs. 7.1.15–7.1.17).
▸ **Polypoidal choroidal vasculopathy (PCV):** PCV is a variation of type 1, or occult, CNV where polyp-shaped abnormal vascular complexes are located underneath the RPE. Large flat, type 1 CNV with multiple PEDs are common findings with PCV. (Figs. 7.1.18–7.1.20).
▸ **Isolated PED:** in the setting of a large, isolated PED, it can sometimes be difficult to determine whether co-existent wet AMD is present even with the aid of a fluorescein angiography (FA).

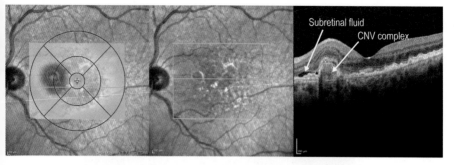

Figure 7.1.1 OCT of classic choroidal neovascularization (far right). Corresponding thickness map (left) and infrared image (middle) are shown.

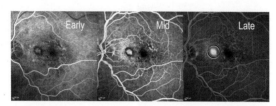

Figure 7.1.2 Fluorescein angiography (corresponding to Figure 7.1.1) shows a well-defined region of hyperfluorescence that is visible in the early frames and grows in intensity in the late frames, but does not enlarge in size, characteristic of classic choroidal neovascularization (red circle).

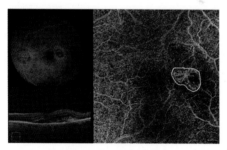

Figure 7.1.3 OCTA *en face* projection image (right) shows classic choroidal neovascularization (surrounding yellow line). Corresponding fluorescein angiography and structural OCT are shown (left).

OCT can help to determine whether overlying intra- or subretinal fluid is present, which would suggest the presence of wet AMD, and OCTA can determine whether vascularization of the PED is present (Fig. 7.1.21).

▸ **Non-exudative CNV:** subclinical, non-leaking choroidal neovascularization may be present in the absence of any signs of clinical exudation such as sub- or intra-retinal fluid. This is termed non-exudative neovascular AMD and has become more apparent with the advent of OCTA (Figs. 7.1.22 and 7.1.23).

OCTA Features: OCTA can confirm the presence of CNV by indirectly imaging vascular flow through the CNV complex. This noninvasive modality can provide intricate details of the internal architecture of the CNV by elucidating its size, location, and branching pattern. Although still an area of great study, differences in CNV subtype can be identified by OCTA. **Type 1 (occult) CNVs** are defined by having a large central or flanking trunk from which emanate numerous smaller vessels in an irregular, radiating pattern (Figs. 7.1.6 and 7.1.7). After treatment, the size of the lesion and vessel density tend not to change much. In contrast, **type 2 (classic) CNVs** tend to show a reduction in lesion size and vessel density following treatment (Figs. 7.1.3 and 7.1.4).

OCTA can be helpful in pinpointing the intraretinal location of **type 3 (retinal angiomatous proliferation) neovascularization** (Fig. 7.1.17). In many cases of neovascular AMD, the CNV is composed of a mixed type, which has become more evident with OCTA. OCTA has also allowed a better understanding of a subclinical, or non-exudative, form of neovascular AMD, whereby a CNV can be visualized on OCTA in the absence of exudative features that are visible clinically or on structural OCT (Figs. 7.1.22 and 7.1.23).

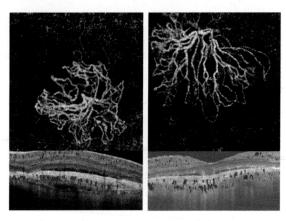

Figure 7.1.4 OCTA *en face* projection images (top) show two separate examples of classic choroidal neovascularization (CNV). Corresponding B-scans (bottom) show the slab segmentation (horizontal red lines), which includes the outer retina and area of CNV located above the retinal pigment epithelium.

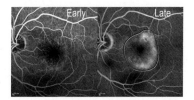

Figure 7.1.5 Fluorescein angiography shows late hyperfluorescence with ill-defined boundaries, which may represent a fibrovascular pigment epithelial detachment, and is characteristic of an occult choroidal neovascularization (within red border).

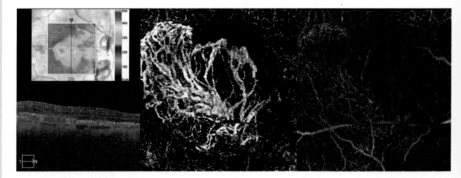

Figure 7.1.6 OCTA *en face* projection (middle) and retina depth encoded (right) images show occult neovascularization localizing to the sub-RPE space. There is a large central trunk with smaller vessels radiating in a configuration resembling a sea fan. Corresponding thickness map and structural OCT are shown (left).

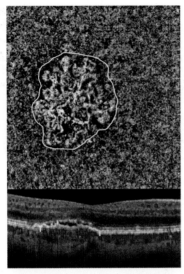

Figure 7.1.7 OCTA *en face* projection (top) and corresponding mid-lesion OCT B-scan (bottom) show occult neovascularization (yellow surrounding line). The slab segmentation is delineated by two horizontal red lines. Within the slab, a vascular flow signal is seen below the level of the RPE (between two yellow lines), corresponding to the area of occult neovascularization.

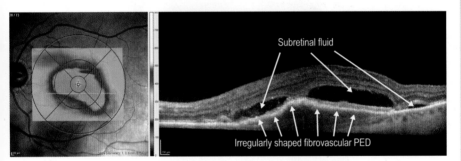

Figure 7.1.8 OCT (corresponding to Figure 7.1.5) of occult choroidal neovascularization (right) and corresponding thickness map (left), pigment epithelial detachment.

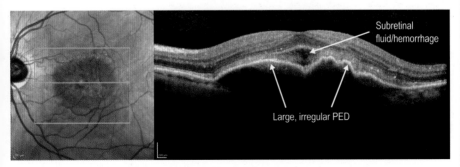

Figure 7.1.9 OCT of choroidal neovascularization with a large, irregular pigment epithelial detachment. The corresponding infrared image is also shown (left).

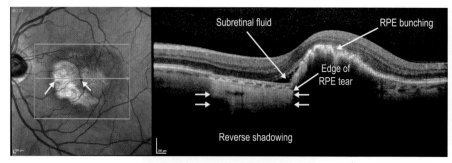

Figure 7.1.10 OCT of the same choroidal neovascularization shown in Figure 7.1.9 one month following treatment with intravitreal anti-VEGF therapy with resultant retinal pigment epithelium (RPE) tear. Due to the absence of the RPE in the region of the tear, reverse shadowing is seen in the deeper structures. The RPE is bunched up where it is still present, blocking deeper structures. There is also still a thin rim of subretinal fluid present. Corresponding infrared image is shown on the left, which helps to visualize the region of the RPE tear.

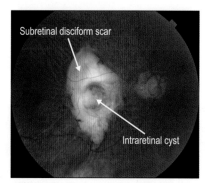

Figure 7.1.11 Color photograph of a subretinal disciform scar that is the result of end-stage wet age-related macular degeneration (AMD). A central intraretinal cyst is present, which is better visualized on OCT.

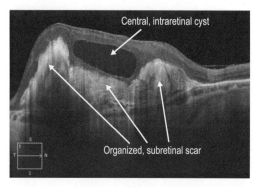

Figure 7.1.12 OCT (corresponding to Figure 7.1.11) shows highly reflective subretinal material corresponding to the organized subretinal scar. A central intraretinal cyst is also present.

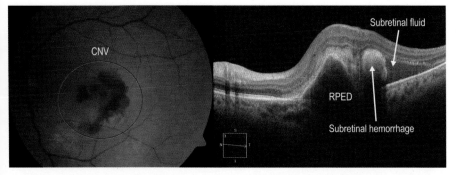

Figure 7.1.13 OCT shows all of the features of wet age-related macular degeneration (AMD) including an irregularly shaped pigment epithelial detachment (PED), subretinal hemorrhage, and subretinal fluid. Subretinal fluid lacks reflectivity on OCT and appears as an empty space, whereas the subretinal hemorrhage has moderate reflectivity and appears as a medium-intensity signal. The corresponding color photograph is shown on the left.

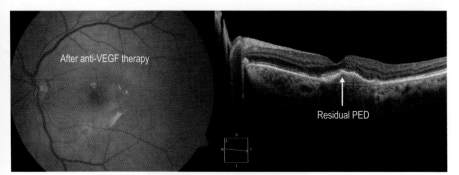

Figure 7.1.14 Following therapy (corresponding to Figure 7.1.13) with numerous intravitreal injections of an anti-vascular endothelial growth factor medication, there was significant improvement in the clinical appearance with resolution of subretinal fluid.

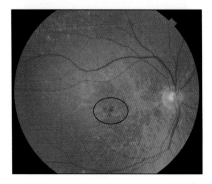

Figure 7.1.15 Color photograph of retinal angiomatous proliferation shows multiple localized intraretinal hemorrhages in an area of retinal thickening.

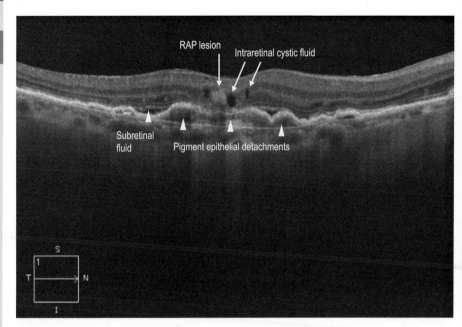

Figure 7.1.16 OCT (corresponding to Figure 7.1.15) shows a hyper-reflective area within the retina, thought to represent the retinal angiomatous proliferation lesion. There is associated intraretinal cystic fluid and underlying subretinal fluid and pigment epithelial detachments.

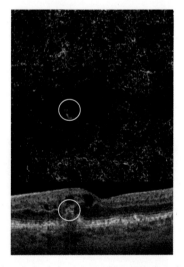

Figure 7.1.17 OCTA *en face* image (top) demonstrates a weak, but abnormal, flow signal (yellow circle) caused by an area of retinal angiomatous proliferation. Corresponding OCT B-scan (bottom) shows an abnormal focal flow signal within the deep retina (yellow circle)

Ancillary Testing: FA is helpful to confirm a diagnosis of wet AMD and for subtyping the lesion (Figs. 7.1.2 and 7.1.5), although this was more useful historically when treatment decisions were based on lesion type. Indocyanine green angiography (ICGA) can help to differentiate less common AMD sub-types that do not respond well to standard anti-VEGF therapy, such as PCV (Fig. 7.1.19).

Treatment: Intravitreal anti-VEGF monotherapy is the mainstay of treatment for most eyes with wet AMD. Current intravitreal treatment options include bevacizumab, ranibizumab, aflibercept, and brolucizumab. PEDs, subretinal fluid, and subretinal hemorrhage often improve or resolve with continued anti-VEGF treatment (Fig. 7.1.14). Idiopathic polypoidal choroidal vasculopathy may be best treated with a combination of focal therapy to the polyps (laser or photodynamic therapy) and anti-VEGF injections.

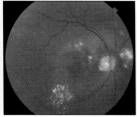 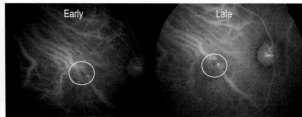

Figure 7.1.18 Color photograph shows multiple subretinal peripapillary polypoidal lesions with associated subretinal fluid and exudate.

Figure 7.1.19 Indocyanine green angiogram shows small, pinpoint hyperfluorescent polyps consistent with a diagnosis of polypoidal choroidal vasculopathy in a patient who responded suboptimally to anti-vascular endothelial growth factor therapy.

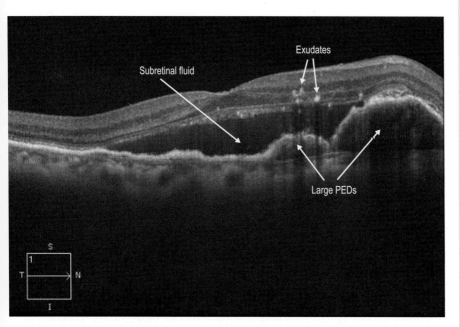

Figure 7.1.20 OCT (corresponding to Figure 7.1.18) shows multiple, large, adjacent PEDs with overlying subretinal fluid. Exudate is also visible as hyper-reflective intraretinal spots.

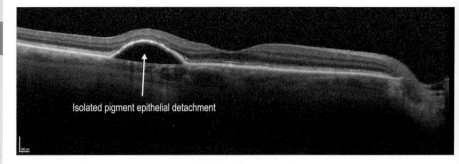

Isolated pigment epithelial detachment

Figure 7.1.21 OCT of an isolated pigment epithelial detachment confirms that there is no associated intraretinal or subretinal fluid in a patient with dry age-related macular dystrophy.

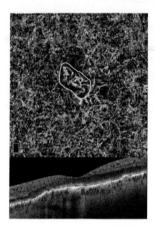

Figure 7.1.22 OCTA *en face* projection (top) of non-exudative neovascular AMD showing type 1 CNV (yellow surrounding line). The corresponding OCT B-scan (bottom) shows vascular flow signal below the level of the RPE.

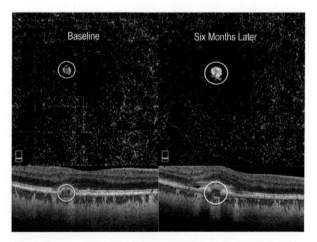

Baseline   Six Months Later

Figure 7.1.23 OCTA of non-exudative neovascular AMD (left) converting to exudative neovascular AMD (right) over time. OCTA *en face* projections (top) show the CNV enlarge over time (yellow to white circle). Corresponding OCT B-scans (bottom) show no exudation at baseline (left) followed by new subretinal hyper-reflective material and subretinal fluid indicative of exudation.

8.1 Posterior Staphyloma

Introduction: Posterior staphyloma occurs in the setting of high myopia (axial length >26 mm) and correlates with its severity. Localized outward protrusions develop as a result of progressive anteroposterior elongation of the globe over time with scleral thinning in the posterior pole.

Clinical Features: Externally, the globe itself may appear elongated, which is consistent with extreme myopia. On fundoscopy, there are associated atrophic changes of the retina, retinal pigment epithelium, and choroid in the posterior pole (Fig. 8.1.1). A teacup-like deformity is present, typically within the macula, but it can also involve the optic nerve. The deformity can be difficult to visualize clinically and requires stereopsis to appreciate. Coexisting pathologies such as atrophic retinal atrophy, epiretinal membrane, macular schisis, macular hole, and vitreomacular traction are common.

OCT Features: OCT is particularly useful to identify posterior staphyloma because of its depth-resolved capability. The appearance of a posterior staphyloma on OCT is rather striking compared with its more subtle clinical appearance. There is loss of the normal horizontal orientation of the retinal layers. In severe cases, OCT reveals significant **posterior bowing and curvature of the posterior eye wall**, including the sclera and overlying choroid and retinal layers (Figs. 8.1.2 and 8.1.3). The choroid is typically almost imperceptible because of significant thinning.

Ancillary Testing: Ultrasonography can be used to document progressive enlargement of the globe and to reveal the posterior out-pouching of the posterior wall of the eye.

Treatment: Treatment of any associated pathology may be required, but no primary therapy for the progressive globe enlargement has been proven to work.

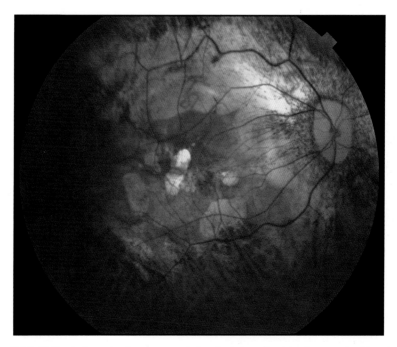

Figure 8.1.1 Color photograph of a severe posterior staphyloma involving the macula. There is extensive retinal pigment epithelium loss, pigmentary changes, and choroidal atrophy present.

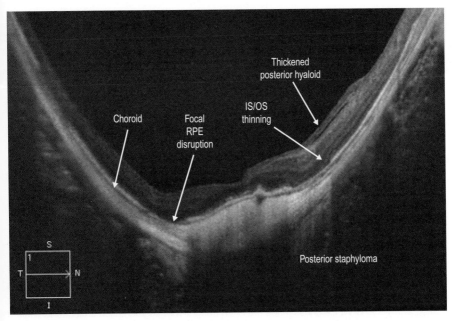

Figure 8.1.2 OCT (corresponding to Figure 8.1.1) of severe posterior staphyloma shows dramatic posterior bowing of the eye wall. The choroid is so thin that it is barely appreciable. The RPE layer has focal disruptions. The retina takes on the same curvature as the sclera. There is also a mild dome-shaped macula present (see Chapter 8.4, Dome-Shaped Macula)

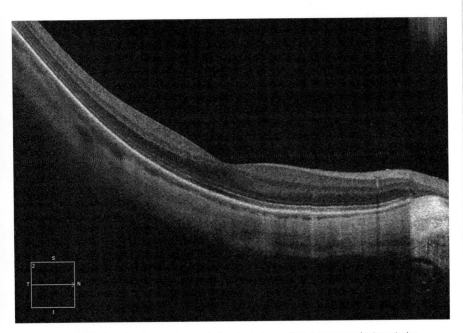

Figure 8.1.3 OCT of moderate macular posterior staphyloma shows more modest posterior curvature compared with Figure 8.1.2.

8.2 | Myopic Choroidal Neovascular Membrane

Introduction: Choroidal neovascularization (CNV) can occur in the setting of pathologic myopia, typically in preexisting areas of Bruch's membrane weakness such as lacquer cracks and chorioretinal atrophy.

Clinical Features: This type of CNV is usually well circumscribed, often pigmented, and occurs in conjunction with a background of typical myopic changes (Figs. 8.2.1 and 8.2.2). Myopic CNV is usually situated within the fovea and is a type 2, or classic, CNV subtype. Its behavior tends to be less aggressive than CNV associated with wet age-related macular degeneration.

OCT Features: Acutely, the CNV complex appears as a well-circumscribed area of **mixed reflectivity** in the subretinal space with overlying sub- and intraretinal fluid (Fig. 8.2.3, inset lower right). Sometimes, the presence of active CNV in high myopia **can be difficult to discern**, even with OCT. In this setting, activity may be recognized by **subtle changes on serial examinations** (Figs. 8.2.4 to 8.2.7). For such comparisons to be accurate, the scans that are taken at different times should be **registered** to assure the exact same region is being imaged over time. In the setting of myopic CNV, thickness maps are often fraught with segmentation artifact and cannot always be relied on to make treatment decisions. OCTA provides a noninvasive modality for visualizing myopic CNV indirectly by detecting blood flow patterns in the macula and choroid, which can be particularly helpful in cases where structural OCT findings are inconclusive. With OCTA, myopic CNV can best be visualized as a net of abnormal vessels on OCTA *en face* images of the deep retinal and choroidal segments (Figs. 8.2.8 and 8.2.9).

Ancillary Testing: Fluorescein angiography (FA) can be helpful to confirm the presence of a type 2 CNV (Fig. 8.2.2).

Treatment: The mainstay of treatment is with intravitreal anti-vascular endothelial growth factor (anti-VEGF) therapy (Fig. 8.2.10), with photodynamic therapy reserved for select cases.

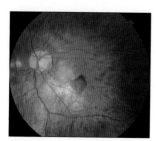

Figure 8.2.1 Color photograph of a myopic CNV shows a well-circumscribed, darkly pigmented submacular lesion involving the inferior fovea.

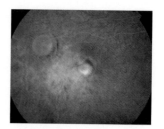

Figure 8.2.2 Fluorescein angiography (late phase, corresponding to Figure 8.2.1) shows a well-circumscribed area of hyperfluorescence consistent with a type 2 CNV.

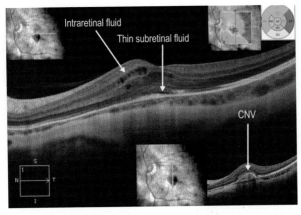

Figure 8.2.3 A horizontal line scan OCT (corresponding to Figure 8.2.1) of the fovea shows thin subretinal fluid with overlying intraretinal fluid at the edge of the lesion. The corresponding thickness map (inset, upper right) helps identify the affected area of thickened retina. A vertical line scan OCT (inset, bottom right) shows an elevated subretinal lesion with mixed reflectivity corresponding to the CNV.

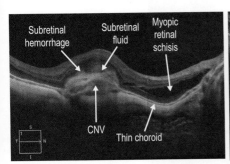

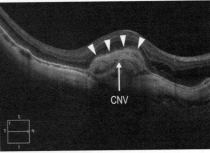

Figure 8.2.4 OCT shows a subretinal dome-shaped hyper-reflective area, which represents a myopic CNV. The distinction of the CNV from the overlying retina is blurred as a result of subretinal hemorrhage and subretinal fluid. These findings are more subtle in a myopic CNV in comparison with other forms of CNV. Characteristic myopic findings including a thin choroid and retinal schisis are also seen.

Figure 8.2.5 OCT (corresponding to Figure 8.2.4) shows a much more distinct border of the retina (arrowheads) and underlying myopic CNV 1 month after treatment with anti-VEGF therapy.

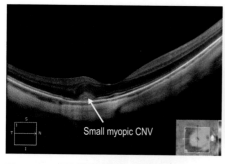

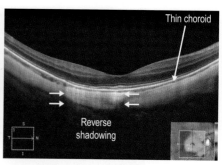

Figure 8.2.6 OCT of a small myopic CNV shows an ill-defined medium reflectivity subretinal elevation that obscures the photoreceptor and ELM layers and has poorly defined edges. (Courtesy Caroline Baumal, MD.)

Figure 8.2.7 OCT (corresponding to Figure 8.2.6) shows complete resolution of the myopic CNV 1 month after treatment with intravitreal bevacizumab. (Courtesy Caroline Baumal, MD.)

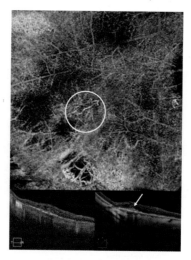

Figure 8.2.8 OCTA *en face* image of the deep retina (top) and structural OCT B-scan with corresponding segmentation lines shows an inactive, small myopic CNV. A localized, tight net of fine vessels represents the CNV on the OCTA image (circle), which corresponds to a hyper-reflective subretinal lesion on structural OCT (arrow).

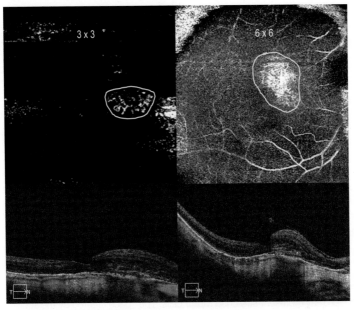

Figure 8.2.9 OCTA *en face* images (3 × 3, left; 6 × 6, right) of active myopic CNV. The fine net of vessels is well visualized (yellow outline).

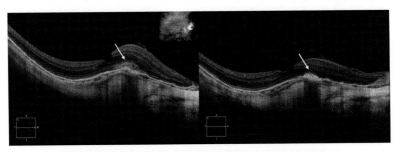

Figure 8.2.10 OCT (corresponding to Figure 8.2.9) at baseline (left) and 1 month after anti-VEGF therapy (right). Note the reduction in CNV size (arrows) following treatment.

8.3 | Myopic Macular Schisis

Introduction: Myopic macular (foveal) schisis is a relatively common finding in eyes with high myopia. The prevalence increases with the degree of myopia. Mild cases do not necessarily impact visual acuity, whereas severe cases usually affect vision. Prior to the advent of OCT, this disorder was significantly under-recognized and poorly described.

Clinical Features: When mild, macular schisis is difficult if not impossible to appreciate fundoscopically. The clinical presence of macular schisis in the setting of high myopia might be presumed based on the presence of other associated features of pathologic myopia such as posterior staphyloma, lacquer cracks, and atrophy. More severe cases can be recognized by diffuse cystic change in the macula and sometimes with concomitant lamellar or full-thickness macular holes.

OCT Features: OCT is critical in confirming the diagnosis and following the morphologic changes in myopic macular schisis. OCT can readily visualize subtle schisis that is often asymptomatic (Fig. 8.3.1), and may be confused for other conditions such as cystoid macular edema. There is a characteristic **splitting of the retinal layers** that tends to occur in the **outer layers**, leaving a thicker inner retina split from a thinner outer retina. Joining these two layers are **perpendicular strands**, which may represent stretched Müller cells. The space created by the schisis is thickest centrally and tapers toward each end. There can be a range of severity in myopic macular schisis, including more moderate (Fig. 8.3.2) and severe (Fig. 8.3.3) changes. The choroid is characteristically thin as in other instances of high myopia. Other changes include prominent posterior hyaloid, epiretinal membrane, lamellar macular hole, or full-thickness macular hole.

Ancillary Testing: Fluorescein angiography is rarely helpful but can be used to rule out myopic choroidal neovascularization. B-scan ultrasonography can reveal some of the features but lacks the resolution of OCT.

Treatment: In mild to moderate cases, no treatment is warranted. However, in severe cases with progressive visual loss, vitrectomy can provide both anatomical and functional improvement.

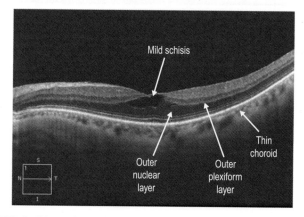

Figure 8.3.1 OCT of mild myopic macular schisis with splitting of the retina at the level of the outer nuclear layer and outer plexiform layer junction.

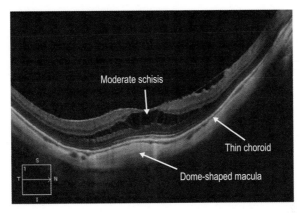

Figure 8.3.2 OCT of moderate myopic macular schisis shows splitting of the retina within the inner portion of the outer nuclear layer. The central area of schisis is thickest with tapering on either side. Three-dimensionally, the schisis space would resemble a flying saucer. Within the schisis cavity, there are perpendicular strands crossing the full length of the cavity, which may represent Müller's cell footplates. Also note that there is a mild posterior staphyloma and dome-shaped macula present. The choroid is also characteristically thin.

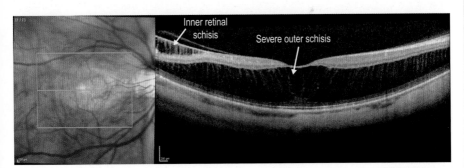

Figure 8.3.3 OCT of severe myopic macular schisis shows dramatic splitting of the retina within the outer nuclear layer. Many perpendicular strands are crossing the schisis cavity. The choroid is almost indiscernible because of significant thinning.

8.4 Dome-Shaped Macula

Introduction: Dome-shaped macula is a rare finding in some highly myopic eyes. It is unclear why certain eyes are affected, but it seems to be a result of localized variations in scleral thickness.

Clinical Features: There is an inward protuberance of the central macula within the larger concave shape of and distinct from a posterior staphyloma in highly myopic eyes. This condition is not appreciated clinically and can only be visualized with OCT. It can be associated with the development of subretinal fluid in the absence of choroidal neovascularization, central serous retinopathy, or other obvious causes.

OCT Features: A **vertical line scan** is more helpful than a horizontal scan in diagnosing dome-shaped macula due to the macular convexity of the dome being more commonly oriented horizontally. Within the convexity of a posterior staphyloma, there is an **inward bowing of the sclera** within the **central macula** (Figs. 8.4.1 and 8.4.2). The overlying macula follows the same contour as the sclera, and there is often a **cap of subretinal fluid** (hyporeflective space) in the absence of any choroidal neovascularization (CNV) or other exudative pathology. The choroid is typically thin, and the underlying sclera can usually be imaged well with standard spectral domain OCT

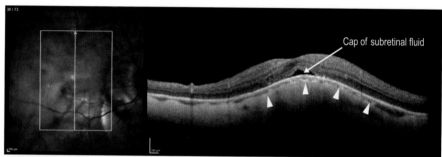

Cap of subretinal fluid

Figure 8.4.1 Vertical OCT line scan in dome-shaped macula shows characteristic inward protuberance of the sclera under the central macula (arrowheads). There is also a cap of hyporeflective subretinal fluid, which is present in the absence of choroidal neovascularization.

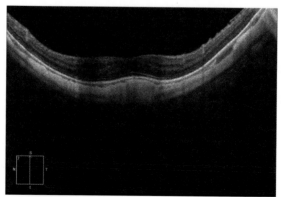

Figure 8.4.2 Vertical OCT line scan in a milder case of dome-shaped macula without a cap of "subretinal fluid."

protocols. However, both enhanced depth and swept source imaging techniques offer the ability to visualize deeper structures and are a better choice for assisting in this diagnosis, if available.

Ancillary Testing: Fluorescein can be helpful to rule out the presence of a concomitant CNV or central serous chorioretinopathy (CSCR).

Treatment: There is no treatment indicated. It is particularly important that, when present, the apparent cap of subretinal fluid is not anti-vascular endothelial growth factor (anti-VEGF) or photodynamic therapy responsive. It should not be considered as proof of the presence of a CNV. A brief anti-VEGF therapeutic trial can be considered but is unlikely to be of benefit.

8.5 | Myopic Tractional Retinal Detachment

Introduction: In the presence of high myopia, a localized tractional retinal detachment within the macula is an uncommon occurrence. The underlying mechanism is not entirely clear, but tractional forces along the vitreoretinal interface related to hyaloidal thickening with partial separation and/or epiretinal membranes are thought to be the predominant factors.

Clinical Features: A localized elevation of the retina, isolated to the macula, is visible clinically in the absence of any peripheral retinal breaks.

OCT Features: The presence of a large neurosensory detachment of the retina, isolated to the macula, is evident (Fig. 8.5.1). Typically, there are associated vitreous membranes with tractional insertions on the detachment. Other pathologic features of high myopia are usually present, such as posterior staphyloma, macular schisis, and/or macular hole.

Ancillary Testing: None.

Treatment: Initial observation may occasionally result in spontaneous release of vitreomacular traction with improvement in the retinal detachment. More commonly, surgical intervention is required with vitrectomy.

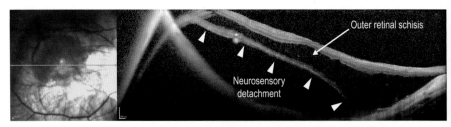

Figure 8.5.1 OCT of a myopic tractional retinal detachment shows a large neurosensory detachment of the retina (arrowheads). There is also significant overlying macular schisis and a posterior staphyloma. Toward the left side of the OCT, there is mirror artifact.

Introduction: Pachychoroid syndrome includes a spectrum of diseases characterized by focal or diffuse increased choroidal thickness (Fig. 9.1.1), with dilated and hyperpermeable choroidal vessels, so-called pachyvessels (Fig. 9.1.2), thinning of overlying choriocapillaris (Fig. 9.1.3), and varying Bruch's membrane and retinal pigment epithelium (RPE) changes. Diseases within the pachychoroid spectrum are central serous chorioretinopathy (CSCR) (see Chapter 12.1), pachychoroid pigment epitheliopathy (PPE), pachychoroid neovasculopathy (PNV), and polypoidal choroidal vasculopathy (PCV). Pachychoroid-associated drusen (pachydrusen) can be found in association with all diseases within the spectrum.

Clinical Features: PPE is thought to be a *forme fruste* of CSCR. It is an asymptomatic condition, often found in the contralateral eye of unilateral CSCR, characterized by reduction of choroidal tessellation on funduscopic examination and small pigment epithelium detachments (PEDs) overlying areas of thickened choroid and/or pachyvessels, in the absence of serous macular detachment.

PNV is characterized by the development of a type 1 macular neovascularization (MNV) in an eye with chronic RPE changes resulting from PPE.

PCV is characterized by the presence of polyps in the choroidal vasculature associated with branching vascular networks (BVN). Clinically, it may present with reddish-orange nodules and exudation associated with serous or hemorrhagic PEDs in the posterior pole, peripapillary area, or peripheral retina. Occurrence of typical drusen is uncommon in this disease, whereas pachydrusen can occur, often associated with increased subfoveal choroidal thickness. Pachydrusen are yellowish deposits that can be found isolated or aggrouped in the posterior pole, peripapillary area, or along vascular arcades.

OCT Features: Diffuse or focal thickening of the choroid are better visualized and measured using either the enhanced depth imaging (EDI) tool on spectral domain OCT (SD-OCT) or a swept source OCT (SS-OCT) device (Fig. 9.1.4). There is no standardized cut-off value to define a thick choroid and the vascular morphology (e.g., presence of pachyvessels) appears to be equally important as the thickness itself to define a pachychoroid.

▸ PPE: OCT in this condition often presents serous PEDs and other mild RPE changes (Fig. 9.1.5), overlying a focal or diffuse thickening of the choroid.
▸ PNV: in addition to diffuse choroidal thickening, focal choroidal vascular dilation might be seen below the neovascular tissue within a PED that corresponds to the type 1 MNV.

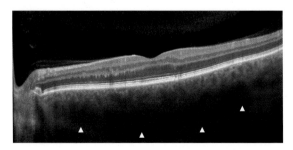

Figure 9.1.1 Spectral domain OCT revealing a diffusely thickened choroid (roughly outlined by white arrowheads).

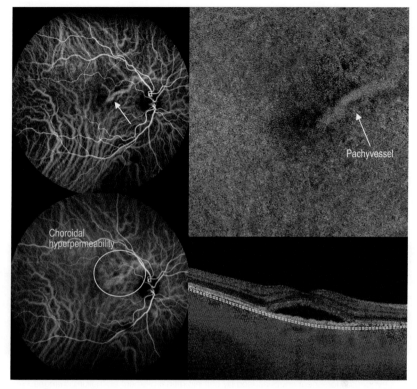

Figure 9.1.2 Indocyanine green angiography (ICGA) (top left, bottom left) of an eye with central serous chorioretinopathy (CSCR), showing a pachyvessel (top left, white arrow) and choroidal hyperpermeability in the macular area (bottom left). *En face* swept-source OCT angiography choriocapillaris slab (top right) revealing the same pachyvessel seen on ICGA. Corresponding B-scan with flow overlay and choriocapillaris segmentation overlaid (bottom right).

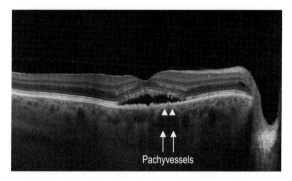

Figure 9.1.3 Spectral domain OCT of an eye with central serous chorioretinopathy, revealing serous retinal detachment and focally thickened choroid, with pachyvessels originated from the Haller's layer, causing thinning of the overlying Sattler's and choriocapillaris layers (white arrowheads).

▶ PCV: characteristic OCT findings of PCV include the presence of abnormal hyper-reflectivity (corresponding to the BVN and polyps) above the Bruch's membrane and below the RPE, and a characteristic "thumb-like" PED corresponding to the location of the polyps (Fig. 9.1.6).

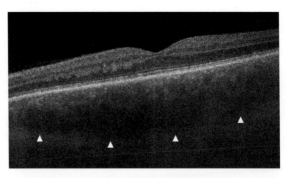

Figure 9.1.4 Swept source OCT revealing a diffusely thickened choroid with a distinct choroidoscleral interface (outlined by white arrowheads).

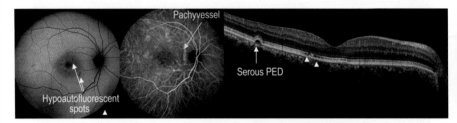

Figure 9.1.5 Pachychoroid pigment epitheliopathy. Fundus autofluorescence (left) showing hypoautofluorescent spots caused by chronic retinal pigment epithelium changes. Hyperautofluorescent changes can also be seen. Indocyanine green angiography (middle) revealing pachyvessels and hyperpermeability. Spectral domain OCT (right) revealing a small serous pigment epithelial detachment and mild outer retina changes (white arrowheads).

A double-layer sign that contains the branching vascular network may be seen associated with the PED (Fig. 9.1.7). In general, OCT angiography (OCTA) provides satisfactory imaging of the BVN. Although the detection rate of polyps with SD-OCTA is lower than with indocyanine green angiography (ICGA) Fig. 9.1.8, data suggest that visualization of polyps with SS-OCTA is quite good.

▶ Pachydrusen: characterized on OCT by homogeneous accumulation of extracellular hyper-reflective material under the RPE, with a clearly demarcated outer border and a more complex shape in comparison with typical soft drusen (Fig. 9.1.9).

Ancillary Testing: On ICGA, increased choroidal permeability can be appreciated in all diseases of the pachychoroid spectrum (Fig. 9.1.1). This test is particularly useful for the diagnosis of PCV, showing a branching vascular network and hypercyanescent polyps (Fig. 9.1.6). Fundus autofluorescence (FAF) presents with chronic RPE disturbance in PPE (Fig. 9.1.5).

Treatment: PPE is an asymptomatic condition that does not require treatment. For both PNV and PCV, treatment options include intravitreal injections of antiangiogenic drugs in monotherapy or in combination with photodynamic therapy. Focal laser therapy may be applied in PCV cases with extrafoveal and peripheral involvement.

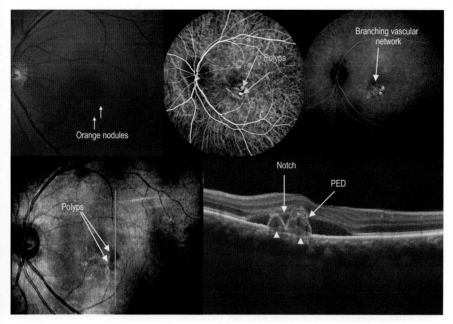

Figure 9.1.6 Color fundus photo (top left) showing orange nodules (white arrows). Indocyanine green angiography (top, middle, and right) showing two polyps (top middle) and a branching vascular network (top right). Spectral domain OCT: Fundus image (bottom left) showing two hyporeflective polyps and B-scan (bottom right) obtained through the polyps showing two epithelial detachments, with a notch, and hyper-reflectivity due to a vascular network above Bruch's membrane (white arrowheads).

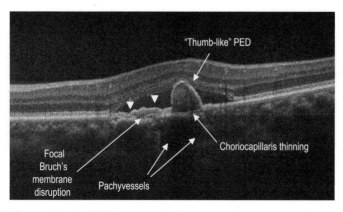

Figure 9.1.7 Spectral domain OCT showing a double-layer sign (white arrowheads) with a focal Bruch's membrane disruption and a "thumb-like" pigment epithelial detachment. Note pachyvessels located at Haller's layer, with thinning of the overlying choriocapillaris.

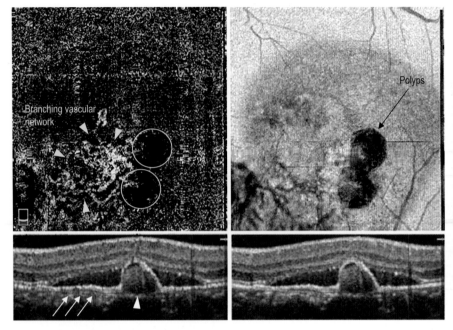

Figure 9.1.8 Spectral domain OCT angiography *en face* (top left) revealing a branching vascular network (BVN) (yellow arrowheads), whereas polyps are not visualized (yellow circles). Correlated B-scan (bottom left) shows a pigment epithelium detachment with underlying flow overlay, corresponding to the BVN (white arrows), but not inside the polyp (white arrowhead). *En face* OCT (top right) revealing reduced signal in the topography of the polyps (black arrow), that can be attributed to shadowing.

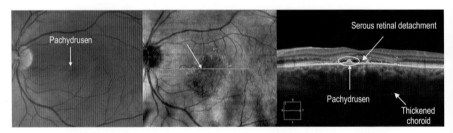

Figure 9.1.9 Color fundus photo showing a pachydrusen (left), also seen on spectral domain OCT, fundus image (middle, white arrow) and B-scan (right, white arrow), in which the pachydrusen is associated to serous retinal detachment and a thickened choroid.

9.2 | Vitreomacular Adhesion and Vitreomacular Traction

Introduction: Vitreomacular adhesion (VMA) is an OCT finding. It represents a perifoveolar detachment of the cortical vitreous from the underlying retina with part of the vitreous remaining attached at the macula and elsewhere in the eye. The underlying macular retina is normal. It is almost always a normal finding, representing the initial evolution of a normal posterior vitreous detachment. Vitreomacular traction (VMT) is present when perifoveolar vitreous detachment is accompanied by retinal morphological changes arising from traction of the vitreous on the retina. There is no known racial predilection for VMT. VMT is more common in women (about 65%), with most patients in their 60s or 70s.

Clinical Features: Patients may complain of decreased central vision with metamorphopsia. On examination, there may be preretinal fibrosis, epiretinal membrane formation, and blunting or alteration of the foveal reflex with a pseudo-hole appearance.

OCT Diagnosis: OCT is the diagnostic modality of choice for both of these entities. In fact, VMA can *only* be reliably diagnosed via OCT. In VMA, OCT shows vitreous separating from around the macula with **persisting adhesion at the macular center**, often in a concentric fashion (Fig. 9.2.1). VMT is accompanied by changes in the retina including **cystic changes**, **macular schisis**, defined as a separation between the outer nuclear and the outer plexiform layer, **epiretinal membrane formation**, and **tractional retinal detachment** (Figs. 9.2.2–9.2.5) The posterior hyaloid often appears **abnormally thickened** in VMT.

Ancillary Testing: A diagnosis of VMT is best made via OCT. Fluorescein angiography may show leakage in a cystic pattern. B-scan ultrasound may demonstrate peripheral detached vitreous but with attachment still noted over the posterior pole.

Treatment: VMA should be observed. The term "symptomatic VMA" will always appear as VMT on OCT. Mild VMT is typically observed. Surgery via vitrectomy or pharmacologic intervention can be considered for eyes with poor or worsening vision.

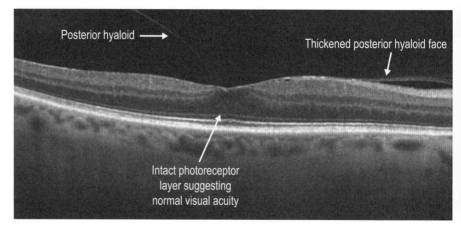

Figure 9.2.1 Vitreomacular adhesion. Note the dense posterior hyaloid face (arrows). The retina appears to be normal.

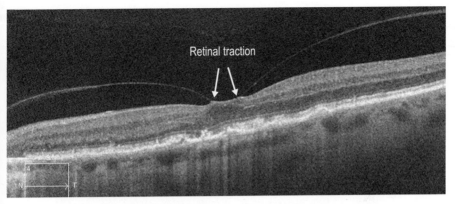

Figure 9.2.2 Early vitreomacular traction. The OCT shows an adherent vitreoretinal interface with retinal changes.

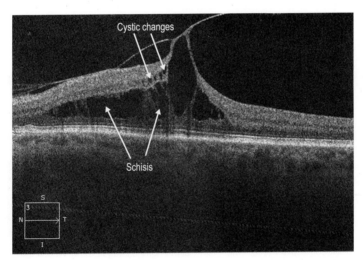

Figure 9.2.3 Vitreomacular traction with macular schisis and outer retinal cystic changes.

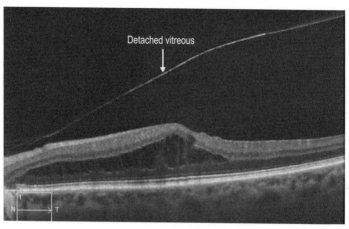

Figure 9.2.4 Vitreomacular traction post-treatment with ocriplasmin showing detachment of the vitreous over the macula (arrow) and improvement of the macular schisis.

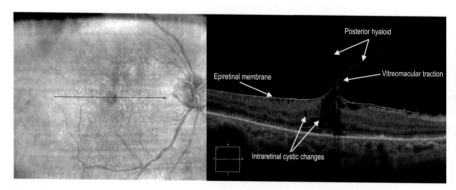

Figure 9.2.5 Vitreomacular traction with epiretinal membrane (stage 3 or 4). Notice the distortion of the foveal surface, disrupted retinal layers, and the intraretinal cystic changes (arrows).

9.3 | Full-Thickness Macular Hole

Introduction: A macular hole is a full-thickness defect in the neurosensory retina occurring at the macular center, usually associated with a central scotoma and decreased vision. Macular holes can be primary (formerly referred to as idiopathic), resulting from vitreomacular traction (VMT) in the course of anomalous posterior vitreous detachment. Primary macular holes are more common in women, most often seen in the sixth or seventh decade of life. Primary macular holes may be bilateral in 10–20% of cases. Secondary macular holes are due to forces other than VMT. They can be traumatic, associated with posterior staphylomas in severe myopia, epiretinal membrane, cystoid macular edema, or rarely associated with solar retinopathy.

Clinical Features: Classic symptoms are acute unilateral decreased vision and occasional metamorphopsia. VMT, formerly sometimes called stage 1 macular hole or impending macular hole, may be seen as a loss of the normal foveolar depression with a yellow spot or ring in the center of the macula. A full-thickness macular hole (FTMH) is seen as a well demarcated, round red spot in the center of the macula surrounded by a grey halo that represents a cuff of subretinal fluid around the hole (Fig. 9.3.1). An operculum may be seen above the hole. Yellowish deposits may be seen within the hole.

Macular holes were classified according to their clinical findings. However, with OCT data available, this classification system is now in flux. This is described in some detail in the following section.

OCT Features: OCT features of macular holes include a **full-thickness defect** in the neurosensory retina (Figs. 9.3.2 to 9.3.5). There may be **cysts** in the neurosensory retina surrounding the area of the hole. A cuff of **subretinal fluid** may be seen around the defect in the retina. The vitreous may be attached to the hole with **vitreomacular traction** or there may be an **operculum** seen in the posterior vitreous on OCT scanning. Chronic macular holes may show loss of the cuff of subretinal fluid. There may also be **RPE atrophy** seen in chronic holes.

OCT-based macular hole classification is based on the size of the hole and the status of the vitreomacular interface:

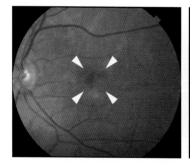 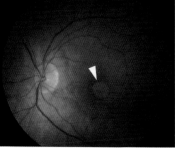

Figure 9.3.1 Fundus photograph of a full-thickness macular hole. The picture to the left shows an acute hole, whereas the one on the right shows a chronic hole with retinal pigment epithelium changes at the margin.

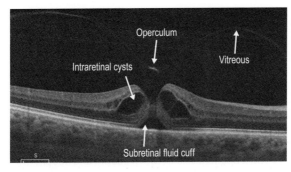

Figure 9.3.2 OCT scan through an acute macular hole showing intraretinal cysts, a cuff of subretinal fluid, and an operculum. Note that the vitreous is detached from the fovea.

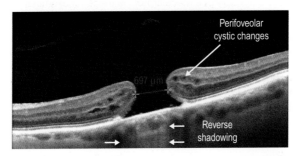

Figure 9.3.3 A large macular hole with the calipers showing a measurement of over 600 μm.

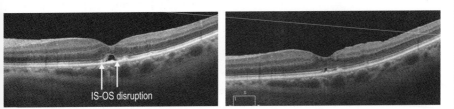

Figure 9.3.4 One week (left) and 1 month (right) post-vitrectomy for macular hole closure. Note the small area of subretinal elevation that decreases with time with restoration of the external limiting membrane (ELM) and a small area of disruption in the IS–OS/ellipsoid layer, or ellipsoid zone (EZ). Various studies have shown that disruption in the ELM, EZ, and the length of disruption of the cone outer segment tips correlates with level of postoperative visual acuity.

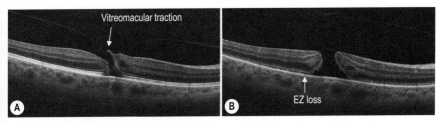

Figure 9.3.5 (A and B) Pre- and postoperative images from a full-thickness macular hole treated with Ocriplasmin (Jetrea). There is resolution of the vitreomacular traction (VMT), but the hole persists and there is loss of the ellipsoid zone (EZ) layer noted (arrows).

▸ **Stage 0 macular hole:** On OCT, this is an eye with vitreomacular adhesion (VMA), which has a FTMH in the contralateral eye. The risk of progression to a full-thickness hole in the eye with VMA may be close to 40%.

▸ **Stage 1 macular hole:** This is VMT.

▸ **Stage 2, 3 and 4 macular holes** per Gass' classification are now reclassified as small, medium, or large macular holes with (stage 4) or without (stages 2 and 3) release of the VMA.

FTMHs are now better classified according to their aperture size on OCT scanning as measured by the caliper function of the OCT scanner:

▸ **Small FTMH:** aperture size less than or equal to 250 µm

▸ **Medium-sized FTMH:** aperture size between 250 µm and 400 µm

▸ **Large FTMH:** aperture size greater than 400 µm

FTMH may further be subclassified by the presence or absence of ongoing VMT.

Ancillary Testing: The diagnosis of a macular hole is made on examination and OCT scanning. Additional tests are usually not warranted.

Management: For stage 0 and 1 macular holes, the management is as described in the VMA/VMT section (Chapter 9.2). FTMHs are typically treated surgically, with excellent prognosis for closure and visual recovery for small and intermediate sized holes. Chronic (>2 years) holes show slightly lower closure rate with surgery, but the visual results are significantly less than acute FTMH. Small and medium-sized FTMH can be treated with intravitreal ocriplasmin with closure rates of approximately 50%.

9.4 | Lamellar Macular Hole

Introduction: A lamellar macular hole (LMH) is a partial-thickness defect characterized by dehiscence of the inner foveal retina from the outer retina, leading to irregular foveal contour but often preserving the photoreceptor layer. Nevertheless, LMH can partially reduce vision. A variety of causes, including abortive full-thickness macular hole (FTMH), vitreomacular traction, or epiretinal membrane formation, can lead to LMH.

Clinical Features: LMH present with symptoms similar to those found in other vitreoretinal interface syndromes, including decreased visual acuity, metamorphopsia, and central scotoma. On examination, LMH can be differentiated from FTMH as a bi- or trilobulated red macular lesion as opposed to a round red spot. Furthermore, their edge is thin compared with the elevated edge of a FTMH caused by subretinal fluid.

OCT Features: OCT features of LMH include a **partial-thickness defect, irregular foveal contour, and separation of the inner and outer retinal layers** (Figs. 9.4.1 to 9.4.3). LMHs are often associated with an **epiretinal membrane** (Figs. 9.4.1 and 9.4.2). LMHs can be distinguished from a macular "pseudohole," which is associated with epiretinal membrane (ERM) traction, by the loss of foveal tissue in the former. There may be **schisis-like changes** or **intraretinal cysts** surrounding the area of the hole (Fig. 9.4.3).

Ancillary Testing: The diagnosis of LMH is made on examination and with OCT scanning. Additional tests are not usually warranted.

Management: LMH typically remain stable over time and may be observed without treatment. However, LMH can rarely progress to FTMH and thus should be monitored.

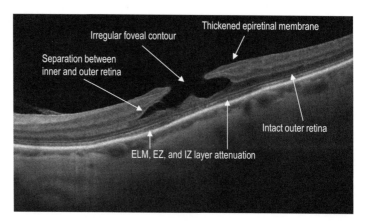

Figure 9.4.1 OCT scan through a lamellar macular hole showing an irregular, anvil-shaped foveal contour and separation of the inner and outer retinal layers. ELM, external limiting membrane; EZ, ellipsoid zone; IZ, interdigitation zone.

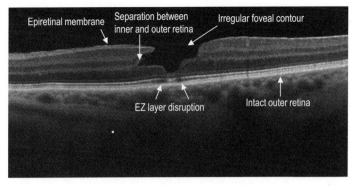

Figure 9.4.2 Lamellar macular hole (LMH) demonstrating foveal EZ disruption.

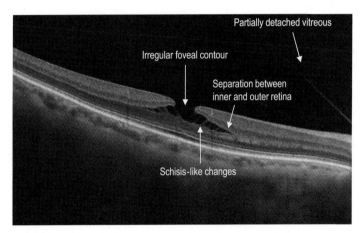

Figure 9.4.3 LMH with schisis-like changes in the inner retina.

9.5 | Epiretinal Membrane

Introduction: Epiretinal membrane (ERM) is common, affecting 6% of patients over 60 years of age. It most commonly develops as a result of vitreoschisis after posterior vitreous detachment or is associated with retinal tears and breaks, cryopexy, previous retinal laser, intraocular surgery, uveitis, or a history of trauma.

Clinical Features: Patients may be asymptomatic or complain of metamorphopsia and blurring of varying severity. On examination, the epiretinal layer can be seen as a glistening membrane overlying the fovea, often associated with retinal striae in a radial fashion and macular thickening (Fig. 9.5.1). Contraction of the membranes can also cause retinal vascular distortion. More severe epiretinal membranes can cause loss of the normal foveal reflex and pseudohole formation.

OCT Features: ERM appears as a **highly reflective layer** overlying the inner retina, which may be adherent to the retina throughout the length of the scan or **adherent** for only a portion of the macular region. Depending on the severity of the ERM, **distortion of the inner retina, loss of foveal contour, retinal thickening and irregularity of the retinal surface, subretinal fluid**, and **foveal schisis** may occur (Figs. 9.5.2, 9.5.3, and 9.5.4). **Cystic changes and macular edema** may also develop within the retina (Figs. 9.5.2 and 9.5.5). Occasionally, ERM may be associated with a **pseudohole** configuration, with **disruption** of the inner retina in the region of the "hole" and **separation** between the outer plexiform layer and the outer nuclear layer seen adjacent to the site of the "hole." However, the outer retinal structures are intact, including the inner and outer segments of the photoreceptors.

On OCT angiography (OCTA), ERMs may be characterized by tortuosity of the retinal vasculature.

Ancillary Testing: Fluorescein angiography may highlight distortion of the blood vessels with leakage of blood vessels at the macula.

Treatment: The treatment of epiretinal membranes is either observation or surgery when the ERM starts to affect vision.

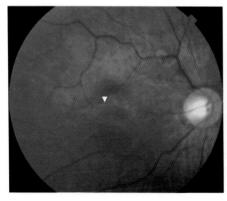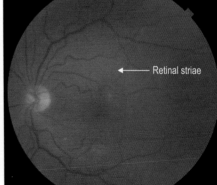

Figure 9.5.1 The photo on the right shows a mild epiretinal membrane (ERM) with retinal striae. The photo on the left shows a denser ERM.

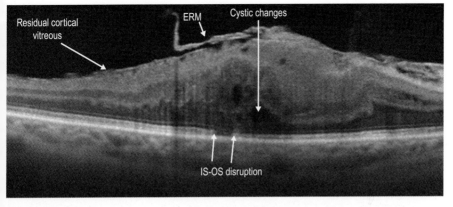

Figure 9.5.2 Denser ERM with macular edema, cystic changes, and distortion in the retinal architecture.

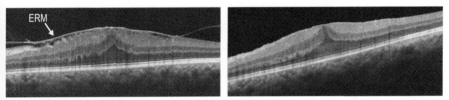

Figure 9.5.3 Preoperative and postoperative OCT scans through an ERM. In the first figure, notice the hyper-reflective membrane causing macular edema. In the second image, the macular thickening is still present but the ERM has been removed.

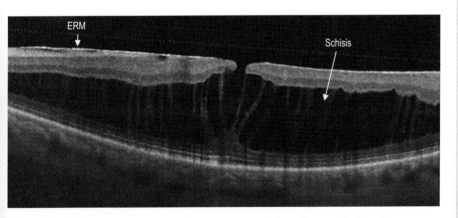

Figure 9.5.4 ERM with traction related schisis. Note the schisis cavities seen in the retina.

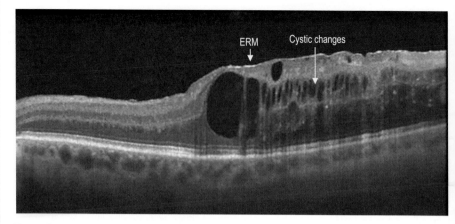

Figure 9.5.5 ERM with macular edema.

10.1 | Postoperative Cystoid Macular Edema

Introduction: Postoperative cystoid macular edema (PCME) is a common cause of vision loss after surgery that can occur following virtually any intraocular procedure, including cataract surgery, vitrectomy, and glaucoma filtering surgery.

Clinical Features: PCME has the characteristic clinical appearance of numerous small cystic cavities bunched together in a petaloid arrangement centered on the fovea (Fig. 10.1.1, left). In some cases, the optic disc will be hyperemic or even frankly edematous. Small flame-shaped superficial hemorrhages in the inner retina are not rare.

OCT Features: The characteristic feature on OCT is **large, hyporeflective cystic spaces** located in the **outer plexiform layer**, although there can also be additional, smaller hypo-reflective spaces within the inner plexiform and nuclear layers (Fig. 10.1.1, right). In more severe cases, there may be a central neurosensory detachment. Following successful treatment, the cystic spaces seen on OCT typically improve (Figs. 10.1.2 and 10.1.3). Eventually, complete resolution of cystoid macular edema (CME) would be expected after adequate treatment.

Ancillary Testing: In all cases, fluorescein angiography reveals PCME, even occasionally when it is not visible clinically or by OCT. The angiographic appearance is very characteristic with late diffuse central leakage in a petaloid pattern (Fig. 10.1.4).

Treatment: PCME is often a self-limited disease, but in visually significant cases various treatments can be used, including topical therapy with corticosteroids and nonsteroidal antiinflammatory drugs, local corticosteroids, anti-vascular endothelial growth factors, or even vitrectomy.

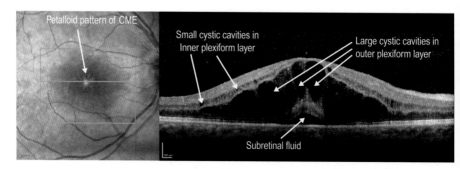

Figure 10.1.1 Infrared image (left) shows a petaloid arrangement of cystic cavities centered on the fovea, characteristic of PCME. OCT (right) shows numerous, hyporeflective cystic cavities located within the outer plexiform layer. There are also smaller hyporeflective cystic cavities located within the inner plexiform and inner nuclear layers. Subretinal fluid is present underneath the fovea. The outer nuclear layer located just above this fluid is hyper-reflective, which is probably an artifact caused by the directional manner by which light traverses the overlying large cystic cavities. (Courtesy Jeffrey S. Heier, MD.)

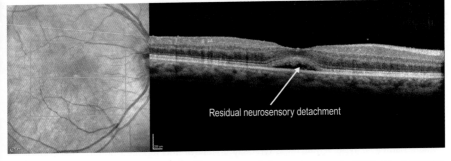

Residual neurosensory detachment

Figure 10.1.2 One month after treatment with topical antiinflammatory agents, OCT shows that the PCME is mostly resolved although a small neurosensory detachment still remains. (Courtesy Jeffrey S. Heier, MD.)

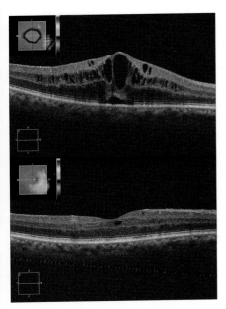

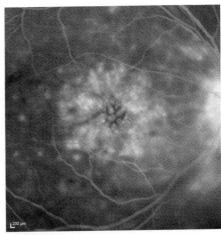

Figure 10.1.3 OCT of PCME showing intraretinal cystic spaces in the outer plexiform, inner plexiform, and inner nuclear layers (top). There is also subretinal fluid in the fovea. After successful treatment with topical steroid, there is near resolution of the cystoid macular edema (CME) except for a small cyst (bottom).

Figure 10.1.4 Fluorescein angiography shows florid late diffuse angiographic leakage in a petaloid pattern. The optic nerve is also leaking, which is not uncommon in severe PCME. (Courtesy Jeffrey S. Heier, MD.)

10.2 Macular Telangiectasia

Introduction: Macular telangiectasia (MacTel) is classified as type 1 or type 2. Type 1 MacTel is considered a form of Coats' disease and is developmental in origin. It is usually unilateral. Type 2 MacTel is an acquired, bilateral disorder that occurs in middle-aged or older adults.

Clinical Features: Type 1 MacTel is typically unilateral and features aneurysmal dilatations of capillaries within the macula. Surrounding exudates are common (Fig. 10.2.1). Type 2 MacTel is typically bilateral and features a loss of the temporal juxtafoveal retinal transparency followed by the development of ectatic capillaries in this region, especially temporally (Fig. 10.2.2). Over time, retinal pigment epithelium (RPE) hyperplasia and pigment deposition may occur with crystal deposits (Fig. 10.2.3).

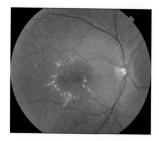

Figure 10.2.1 Color photograph of MacTel type 1 shows numerous aneurysmal abnormalities of varying size within the temporal macula. There is associated retinal thickening and surrounding hard exudate. The fellow macula was normal in appearance.

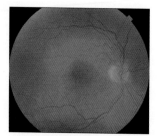

Figure 10.2.2 Color photograph of MacTel type 2 shows loss of the foveal reflex with subtle microaneurysmal abnormalities in the temporal parafoveal region. Fine, crystalline deposits in the same region are barely discernable but could be seen clinically. Similar findings were seen in the fellow eye.

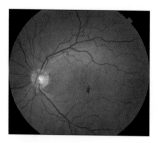

Figure 10.2.3 Color photograph of more advanced MacTel type 2 shows retinal pigment epithelium clumping and hyperplasia with foveal atrophy and obvious crystalline deposits.

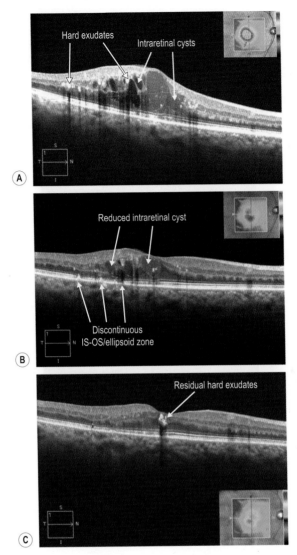

Figure 10.2.4 (A) OCT (corresponding to Figure 10.2.1) in MacTel type 1 shows numerous intraretinal cystic cavities of low and medium reflectivity and small hyper-reflective deposits within the retina, corresponding to hard exudates. (B) OCT 4 months after treatment with focal grid laser shows a significant reduction in the cystoid macular edema and hard exudates. There are multiple discontinuous areas in the IS–OS/ellipsoid zone (arrows), which represent laser scars. (C) OCT 2.5 years after focal laser treatment (no additional treatment was performed) shows resolution of cystoid macular edema with a small amount of residual exudate. The laser scars have faded (arrow).

OCT Features:

▸ MacTel type 1: there is cystoid **intraretinal edema** and subretinal fluid similar in appearance to cystoid macular edema from other etiologies (Fig. 10.2.4).

▸ MacTel type 2: there are **lamellar defects within various layers** of the retina, characteristically starting with involvement of the region just **temporal to the fovea**. These are seen on OCT as irregular, **hyporeflective cavities** (Fig. 10.2.5), which can vary in appearance (Fig. 10.2.6). The region temporal to the fovea is more involved than the nasal region, particularly earlier on in the disease course. With chronic disease, pigment deposition and atrophy may develop

(Fig. 10.2.7). Rarely, secondary, type 3 choroidal neovascularization (CNV) can occur (Fig. 10.2.8). Optical coherence tomography angiography (OCTA) allows more definitive identification of CNV, when present, compared with structural OCT or even fluorescein angiography (FA) (Fig. 10.2.9). OCTA provides the ability to visualize the deep capillary plexus, where there tends to be more disease impact in MacTel type 2 compared with more superficial capillary layers. Abnormal, telangiectatic vessels in the juxtafoveal region are well visualized (Fig. 10.2.10). OCTA serves as an adjunct to structural OCT in the diagnosis and management of MacTel type 2 and it may offer unique insight into its pathophysiology.

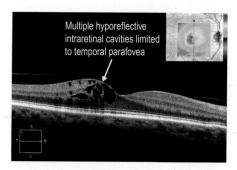

Figure 10.2.5 OCT (corresponding to Figure 10.2.2) in MacTel type 2 shows numerous hyporeflective cavities throughout multiple retinal layers but limited to the temporal parafoveal region.

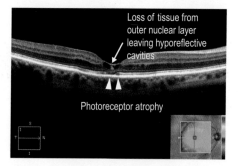

Figure 10.2.6 OCT in MacTel type 2 shows loss of tissue from the outer nuclear layer within the fovea, leaving hyporeflective cystic cavities, more prominent temporally. There is also underlying photoreceptor atrophy (arrowhead).

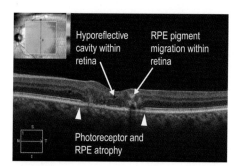

Figure 10.2.7 OCT (corresponding to Figure 10.2.3) in MacTel type 2 shows significant photoreceptor and retinal pigment epithelium (RPE) atrophy (between arrowheads). There is pigment migration from the RPE within the layers of the retina. A small hyporeflective cavity is present within the fovea. The crystalline deposits are not clearly seen.

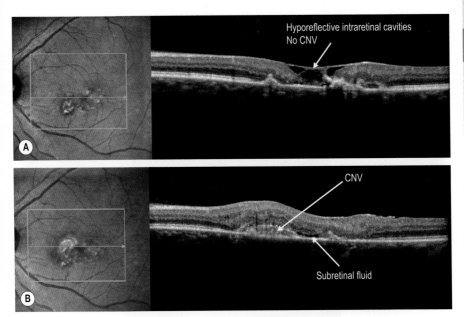

Figure 10.2.8 (A) OCT in MacTel type 2 with characteristic hyporeflective intraretinal cavities involving the fovea, prior to the development of a choroidal neovascularization (CNV). (B) OCT at a later time point shows a CNV with adjacent subretinal fluid, which developed spontaneously.

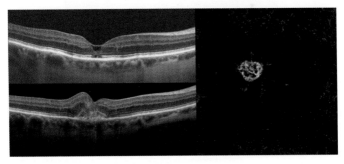

Figure 10.2.9 OCT B-scans of typical MacTel type 2 (top left) with the development of secondary CNV (bottom left). Corresponding OCTA *en face* image (right) shows well defined CNV.

Ancillary Testing: FA can be helpful in both types of MacTel. In MacTel type 1, there are aneurysms of varying size and distribution associated with an abnormal capillary plexus or areas of non-perfusion (Fig. 10.2.11). In MacTel type 2, there are prominent telangiectatic capillaries in the temporal parafoveal region, which leak (Fig. 10.2.12). The cystic changes seen on OCT correspond to leakage on FA. The FA changes may come before or after OCT evidence of the disease is present.

Treatment: MacTel type 1 is treated primarily with focal laser to the telangiectasias. Photodynamic therapy, intravitreal corticosteroids, and anti-vascular endothelial growth factor have all been used with reported success as well. MacTel type 2 has no therapy. Secondary consequences such as choroidal neovascularization or macular hole in type 2 may be successfully treated.

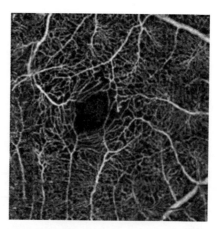

Figure 10.2.10 OCTA *en face* image of MacTel type 2 shows typical features including an irregular foveal avascular zone with telangiectatic changes in the juxtafoveal region with decreased vessel density.

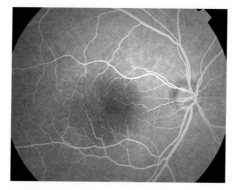

Figure 10.2.11 Fluorescein angiography (FA) (corresponding to Figure 10.2.1) shows numerous hyper-fluorescent aneurysmal capillary dilatations within an abnormal capillary network, most prominent in the temporal parafoveal region.

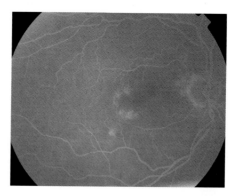

Figure 10.2.12 FA (corresponding to Figure 11.2.2) shows an enlarged foveal avascular zone bordered by leaking capillary abnormalities in the temporal parafoveal region.

10.3 | Uveitis

Introduction: Intermediate and posterior forms of uveitis both commonly affect posterior structures of the eye. Anterior uveitis can also occasionally cause cystoid macular edema (CME).

Clinical Features: Clinical findings vary widely depending on the specific disease state. Common symptoms include decreased vision, floaters, and a red, painful eye. Intraocular inflammation is the key finding. The primary location of intraocular inflammation determines whether anterior, intermediate, or posterior uveitis is present. Optic disc edema and CME may be associated clinical findings.

OCT Features: The presence of **optic disc edema**, **CME**, **subretinal fluid**, and **vitritis** are clinical features of uveitis that can be well visualized with OCT. Active posterior uveitis can lead to optic disc edema, CME, and subretinal fluid (Fig. 10.3.1). OCT is useful in this setting to **monitor for treatment response** (Fig. 10.3.2). Anterior uveitis can also result in isolated CME, which can sometimes be more readily detected on an **OCT thickness map** rather than a line scan (Figs. 10.3.3 and 10.3.6). Pars planitis often leads to significant associated CME (Fig. 10.3.4), which can respond well to treatment with periocular steroids (Fig. 10.3.5). Inflammation within the vitreous cavity can be visualized with OCT if the inflammatory material is near the retinal surface and not significant to the point where the signal intensity is degraded (Figs. 10.3.6 and 10.3.7). Choroidal neovascularization (CNV) can complicate some forms of posterior uveitis (e.g., multifocal choroiditis, sarcoid). Subretinal fluid and even frank exudative retinal detachment can also be seen.

Ancillary Testing: A thorough, focused medical workup is often indicated in the setting of intermediate and posterior uveitis. Referral to a rheumatologist and/or uveitis specialist may be required in more complicated cases.

Treatment: Topical, periocular, and intravitreal steroids are the mainstay of local therapy. Systemic therapy with steroids or immunomodulators may be required via oral and/or intravenous routes.

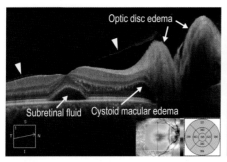

Figure 10.3.1 OCT in a case of sarcoid posterior uveitis. Optic disc edema, cystoid macular edema (CME), and subretinal fluid are present. The posterior hyaloid can be seen (arrowheads). The associated thickness map (inset) artifactually picks up the subretinal fluid as retinal thickness because of an error in the segmentation algorithm, which measures from the retinal pigment epithelium layer instead of the most posterior retina structure.

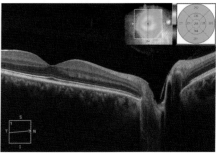

Figure 10.3.2 OCT 3 months after treatment with oral steroids (corresponding to Figure 10.3.1) shows resolution of the optic disc edema, CME, and subretinal fluid. Due to the consistent segmentation error, the associated thickness map (inset) is useful to monitor improvement over time.

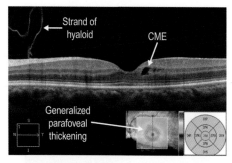

Figure 10.3.3 OCT in a case of sarcoid anterior uveitis shows subtle CME, which was visually symptomatic. The associated thickness map (inset) shows generalized parafoveal thickening, which gives a better overall sense of the CME than the isolated line scan. There is a strand of hyaloid that is visible, which is not of any clinical significance.

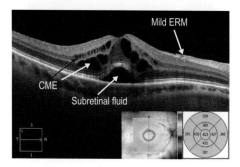

Figure 10.3.4 OCT in a case of pars planitis shows severe CME with associated subretinal fluid. The CME is located within the inner nuclear layer (red arrow) and Henle fiber layer (or axonal outer plexiform layer; white arrow). There is also a mild associated epiretinal membrane (ERM).

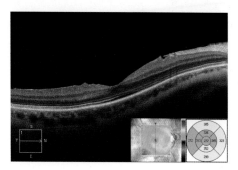

Figure 10.3.5 OCT 1 month after treatment with sub-Tenons triamcinolone (corresponding to Fig. 10.3.4) shows complete resolution of CME and subretinal fluid. The associated thickness map (inset) highlights these changes.

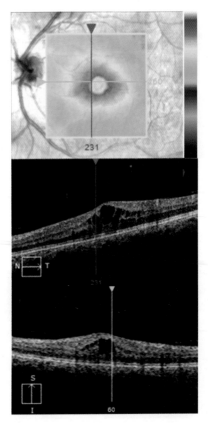

Figure 10.3.6 OCT thickness map (top), horizontal line scan (middle), and vertical line scan (bottom) show active posterior uveitis with CME and numerous hyper-reflective dot-like vitreous opacities corresponding to inflammatory material.

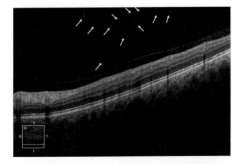

Figure 10.3.7 OCT in active uveitis can visualize even small amounts of inflammation within the vitreous cavity, overlying the retina (arrows).

11.1 | Central Serous Chorioretinopathy

Introduction: Central serous chorioretinopathy is characterized in the acute phase by serous detachment of the retina over one or more areas of leakage from the choroid through a defect in the retinal pigment epithelium (RPE). It is usually self-resolving, but in some cases it can become chronic. Its chronic phase is marked by retinal thinning, cystic retinal degeneration, cystoid macular edema, and diffuse RPE loss. This condition occurs most commonly in men between 20 and 50 years of age. Predisposing factors are type A personality, stressful events, corticosteroid use, and conditions associated with hypercortisolism such as pregnancy and Cushing's syndrome.

Clinical Features: Patients usually present with a unilateral decrease and distortion of central vision. Examination reveals a macular, well-circumscribed neurosensory retinal detachment often with one or more retinal pigment epithelial detachments. Signs of inactive or prior bouts of central serous chorioretinopathy (CSCR) can often be found in the contralateral eye (Fig. 11.1.1).

OCT Features:

▸ **Acute:** the OCT reveals a well-circumscribed neurosensory **retinal detachment** seen as an elevation of the retinal layers with **optically clear fluid** occupying the space between the outer retina and the RPE layer (Fig. 11.1.2). Often (75%) these are also associated with a small **pigment epithelial detachment**, seen as elevation of the RPE layer with underlying shadowing. The retina may sometimes be **thickened** in the acute phase. Choroidal thickening is almost universally present when compared to normal as well as to fellow eyes in acute CSCR, and this may be better visualized using the enhanced depth imaging (EDI) protocol on most commercial OCT scanners. This **diffuse thickening** may be seen to improve when the acute phase of the CSCR resolves.

▸ **Chronic** CSCR may be accompanied by accumulation of hyper-reflective material in the subretinal space (Fig. 11.1.3). Cystic retinal changes and eventual retinal thinning has been reported overlying the areas of subretinal fluid in chronic CSCR. This may be accompanied by photoreceptor and RPE loss. The loss of photoreceptors on OCT may also be associated with decreased best corrected visual acuity even after resolution of subretinal fluid.

▸ **Multifocal** CSCR is characterized by multiple discrete areas of neurosensory detachments. As the CSCR resolves, the subretinal fluid is seen to decrease and then disappear. Quantitative OCT measurements of subretinal fluid are useful in monitoring for improvement and resolution.

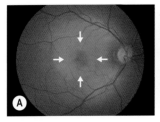 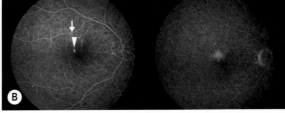

Figure 11.1.1 (A) Fundus photo showing a discrete, well-circumscribed elevation at the macula (arrows). (B) Fluorescein angiography in the early phase shows an area of hyperfluorescence (arrowhead) with leakage noted in the late phase. Note the adjacent areas of hyperfluorescence (arrow) indicative of retinal pigment epithelium window defects characteristically seen in patients with central serous chorioretinopathy.

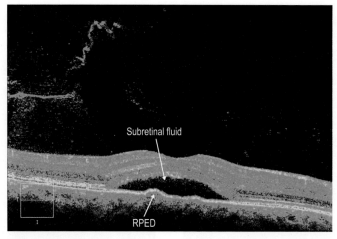

Figure 11.1.2 OCT scanning shows a neurosensory retinal detachment. A small retinal pigment epithelial detachment can sometimes be visualized.

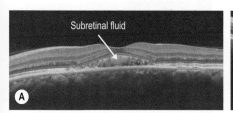
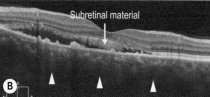

Figure 11.1.3 (A) Chronic central serous chorioretinopathy. Note the subretinal material accumulation and the change in reflectivity of the outer nuclear layer on OCT. (B) Enhanced depth imaging of chronic central serous chorioretinopathy (CSCR). Note that the bottom of the choroid cannot be visualized because of choroidal thickening (arrowheads). There is accumulation of subretinal material.

OCTA Features: OCTA is helpful in the detection of choroidal neovascularization (CNV), a relatively uncommon complication in CSCR but one that requires prompt intervention. OCTA has the ability to provide detailed structural information of the CNV and has the advantage of not being impeded by staining or choroidal leakage as seen in dye-based angiography (Fig. 11.1.4).

Ancillary Testing: Fluorescein angiography shows one or more focal leaks at the RPE level with subretinal pooling of dye. Although indocyanine green angiography is not usually necessary to make the diagnosis, it reveals large hyperfluorescent patches with late leakage. Fundus autofluorescence may show patchy areas of hyper-autofluorescence in the macular area.

Treatment: Most cases of CSCR resolve spontaneously within 4–6 months with improvement of visual acuity. Occasionally, therapeutic options such as focal laser to the leaking spot (if it is extrafoveal) or photodynamic therapy may be useful to expedite resolution or in chronic CSCR.

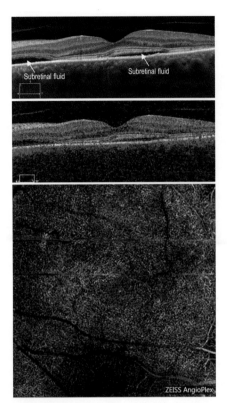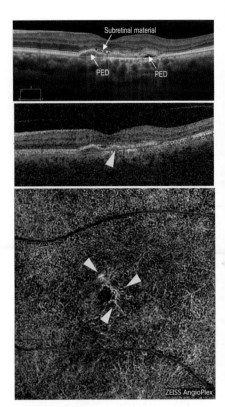

Figure 11.1.4 A case of central serous chorioretinopathy (CSCR) without evidence of choroidal neovascularization (CNV) is shown on the left side panel, and a CSCR case with CNV on the right side panel. Structural B-scans (middle images) show subretinal and sub RPE fluid/material (arrows), and the OCTA flow overlay co-registered with the B-scan provides useful information indicating presence of perfusion on the righthand B-scan (arrowhead). The CNV can be visualized as loops or tufts of irregular blood vessels on enface OCTA scan of the avascular retina slab (bottom images; arrowheads).

11.2 | Hydroxychloroquine Toxicity

Introduction: Retinal toxicity from hydroxychloroquine is rare, especially when dosed appropriately (≤5 mg/kg of real weight/day is recommended). After 5 years of use, the incidence of toxicity is about 1% and increases with additive use over time. Major risk factors for toxicity include excessive daily dosage, renal disease, and concomitant tamoxifen use.

Clinical Features: The findings of hydroxychloroquine retinopathy, even in early and moderate disease, can be clinically silent. Later in the disease, there is a bull's eye maculopathy that becomes evident (Fig. 11.2.1).

OCT Features: OCT is one of the most useful and sensitive diagnostic tests for identifying retinal toxicity caused by hydroxychloroquine. Findings in early disease can be very subtle and may be easier to visualize on a retinal thickness map (Fig. 11.2.2). The earliest signs include subtle parafoveal outer retinal thinning with loss of the cone outer segment tip line. Disease appears in the temporal macula prior to the nasal macula. In moderate disease, there is more obvious **thinning of the outer retinal layers** in a **parafoveal** distribution including loss of the **retinal pigment epithelium** (RPE) **and IS/OS/ellipsoid zone** (Fig. 11.2.3). With advanced disease, there can be profound outer retinal layer loss in a **parafoveal wreath pattern** leading to the so-called "**flying saucer-like" appearance** (Fig. 11.2.4). The **central fovea is characteristically preserved**, even in advanced disease. Although disease burden tends to affect both eyes symmetrically, there can be more severe disease impact in one eye (Fig. 11.2.5).

Ancillary Testing: Multifocal electroretinogram testing is helpful in early or borderline cases to detect subtle abnormalities in central visual function. Fundus autofluorescence and central visual field testing (10–2) are also helpful as adjunctive tests.

Treatment: Stopping hydroxychloroquine at the earliest sign of retinal toxicity is crucial. Retinopathy is irreversible and retinal toxicity may be progressive even after discontinuation of hydroxychloroquine.

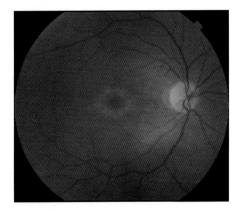

Figure 11.2.1 Color photograph of advanced hydroxychloroquine retinopathy with a classic bull's eye maculopathy.

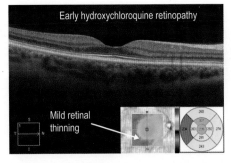

Figure 11.2.2 OCT in a patient with very early hydroxychloroquine retinopathy shows an essentially normal line scan. The key finding is on the thickness map (inset), which reveals mild retinal thinning in a parafoveal pattern, more in the temporal macula.

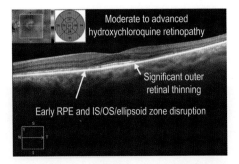

Figure 11.2.3 OCT in a patient with moderate to advanced hydroxychloroquine retinopathy shows fairly extensive outer retinal thinning with loss of the retinal pigment epithelium (RPE) and IS/OS/ellipsoid zone, particularly temporally (right of arrowhead). There is also outer retinal loss to a milder degree in the nasal macula with early RPE and IS/OS/ellipsoid zone disruption. The corresponding thickness map (inset) nicely illustrates the degree of overall thinning.

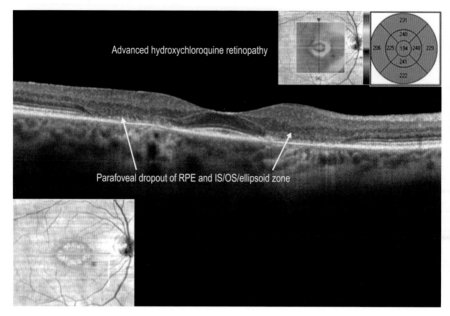

Figure 11.2.4 OCT in a patient with advanced hydroxychloroquine retinopathy (corresponding to Fig. 11.2.1) shows outer retinal thinning with abrupt dropout of the RPE and IS/OS/ellipsoid zone in a parafoveal ring (between arrowheads). There is a classic "flying saucer" appearance created by preservation of the central fovea. The bull's eye maculopathy is seen on the corresponding OCT image (inset, left), and the degree of overall thinning is seen on the corresponding thickness map (inset, right).

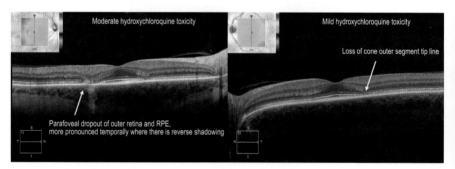

Figure 11.2.5 OCT in a patient with asymmetric hydroxychloroquine retinopathy. The right eye exhibits moderate toxicity while the left eye exhibits mild toxicity.

11.3 | Pattern Dystrophy

Introduction: Pattern dystrophies encompass a group of phenotypically similar macular disorders that are inheritable and share a common genetic defect in the PRPH2 gene. They are usually inherited in an autosomal dominant pattern.

Clinical Features: There are dark, yellow, and/or orange pigment disturbances at the level of the retinal pigment epithelium (RPE), leading to characteristic patterns of deposition in the central macula, which are often vitelliform-like (Fig. 11.3.1). There is a lifetime risk up to 18% of developing secondary choroidal neovascularization (CNV). The clinical features are usually symmetric, but there can be heterogeneity between eyes (Fig. 11.3.2).

OCT Features: A disturbance at the **level of the RPE** is the rule. In the setting of a **vitelliform-like lesion**, there is moderately reflective material underneath or within the RPE layer (Fig. 11.3.3). Below this are highly reflective, drusen-like deposits. In the absence of a vitelliform-like lesion, there are typically **highly reflective, drusen-like deposits** within the RPE layer (Fig. 11.3.4). There can be a **hyporeflective, empty space** overlying the pigmentary disturbance. The significance of this fluid-like compartment is not clearly understood, but it usually does not represent the presence of choroidal neovascularization and would not be expected to be vascular endothelial growth factor (VEGF)-responsive. OCTA can be helpful in identifying the occurrence of secondary CNV (Fig. 11.3.5).

Ancillary Testing: Fluorescein angiography and OCTA can be helpful in ruling out secondary choroidal neovascularization, particularly when OCT reveals the presence of a fluid-like subretinal compartment. Fundus autofluorescence often has a characteristic appearance that can aid in the diagnosis (Fig. 11.3.6).

Treatment: No treatment is available, unless there is secondary choroidal neovascularization, which is treated with intravitreal anti-VEGF therapy.

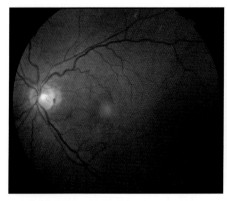 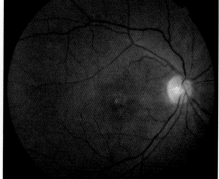

Figure 11.3.1 Color fundus photograph shows a yellowish, circular vitelliform-like lesion within the central macula.

Figure 11.3.2 Color fundus photograph of fellow eye from Figure 11.3.1 shows numerous clumps of pigment within the central macula. This probably represents a collapsed vitelliform lesion.

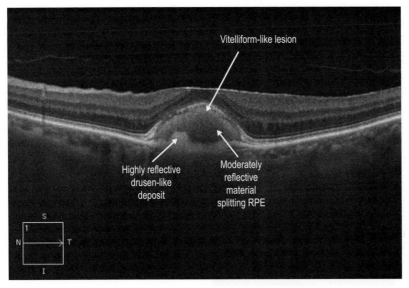

Figure 11.3.3 OCT (corresponding to Figure 11.3.1) shows moderately reflective material that appears to split the RPE layer. There are also highly reflective, drusen-like deposits underlying this area.

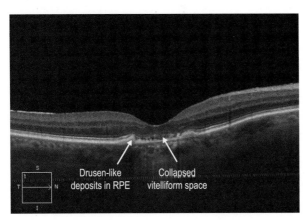

Figure 11.3.4 OCT (corresponding to Figure 11.3.2) shows highly reflective, drusen-like deposits corresponding to the pigment disturbances seen in the color photograph.

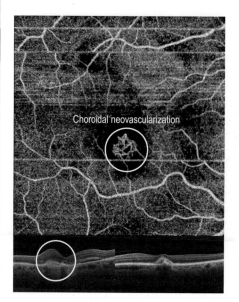

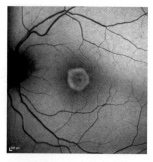

Figure 11.3.6 Fundus autofluorescence shows a well-circumscribed, circular area of hyperautofluorescence with intermingled, splotchy, small areas of hypoautofluorescence.

Figure 11.3.5 OCTA shows secondary CNV (circle) that developed in the setting of pattern dystrophy. Fellow eye OCT (bottom right) shows typical features of pattern dystrophy.

11.4 | Oculocutaneous Albinism

Introduction: Oculocutaneous albinism is a rare, typically autosomal recessive disorder featuring dysfunction of the melanin-producing cells in the eye, hair, and skin. Tyrosinase-negative forms feature an inability to produce melanin, whereas tyrosinase-positive forms have a decreased ability to produce melanin.

Clinical Features: The fundus of tyrosinase-negative individuals has a complete lack of pigmentation, whereas tyrosinase-positive individuals have a variable, but reduced, amount of fundus pigmentation (Fig. 11.4.1). Foveal hypoplasia is characteristically present in both types.

OCT Features: OCT line scans of the central macula reveal **lack of a distinguished foveal depression**, evidence of foveal hypoplasia (Fig. 11.4.2). As a result of this, the corresponding thickness map shows central thickening in comparison with the normative database.

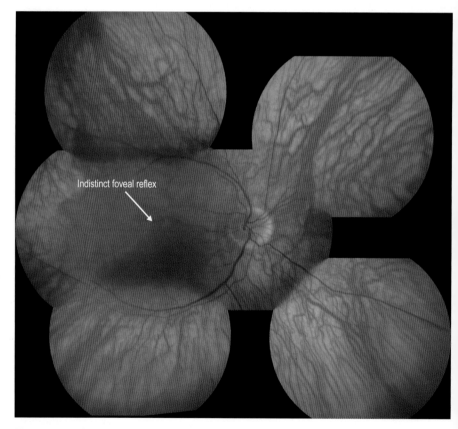

Indistinct foveal reflex

Figure 11.4.1 Color photograph of a patient with tyrosinase-positive oculocutaneous albinism shows a blond fundus with no distinct fovea.

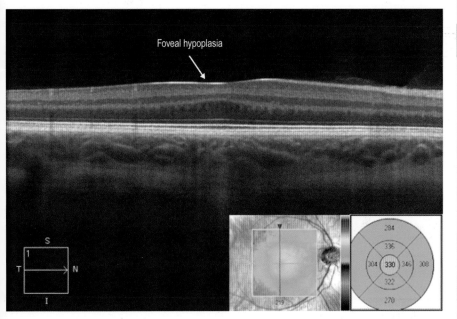

Figure 11.4.2 OCT line scan (corresponding to Figure 11.4.1) through the central macula shows foveal hypoplasia with lack of a well-defined foveal depression. The accompanying thickness map (inset) shows increased thickness centrally in comparison with a normative database due to the lack of a normal foveal depression.

Ancillary Testing: Abnormal decussation of temporal nerve fibers is a characteristic feature seen on visually evoked cortical potential testing. Genetic testing can be performed for mutations in the four genes (TYR, OCA2, TYRP1, or SLC45A2), which, when defective, cause different forms of the disease.

Treatment: Chediak–Higashi and Hermansky–Pudlak syndromes are associated with oculocutaneous syndrome and can be lethal. Frequent infections may be seen in Chediak–Higashi syndrome, and easy bruising can be seen in Hermansky–Pudlak syndrome. Prompt hematologic consultation should be made if either of these syndromes is suspected.

11.5 | Subretinal Perfluorocarbon

Introduction: Perfluorocarbon (PFC) liquid is a dense, clear synthetic liquid used as an intraoperative adjunct during vitrectomy primarily to assist in the repair of complex retinal detachments. PFC liquid can inadvertently migrate into the subretinal space, which may only be identified postoperatively. The risk may be higher with smaller gauge vitrectomy systems.

Clinical Features: Subretinal PFC liquid appears as a localized spherical elevation of the retina (Fig. 11.5.1). The location of the subretinal PFC depends on how the PFC made its way under the retina intraoperatively. If the macula is involved, central visual acuity can be adversely affected.

OCT Features: OCT through a subretinal PFC liquid droplet reveals a **hyporeflective cavity** similar in density to the vitreous space (Fig. 11.5.2). The overlying retina is thin due to a mechanical effect of the dense liquid. Sometimes it can appear as if the PFC liquid is within the retina although it is actually underneath (Fig. 11.5.3).

Ancillary Testing: None.

Treatment: If the PFC liquid is under the macula and affecting visual acuity, it can be removed (Fig. 11.5.4). This requires performing a vitrectomy and using a small-gauge cannula (i.e., 41 G) to create an access retinotomy for direct drainage.

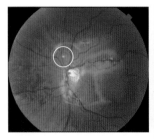

Figure 11.5.1 Color photograph of a retained subretinal PFC liquid droplet superonasal to the optic nerve (circle) following repair of a complex retinal detachment with a giant retinal tear and silicone oil tamponade. (Courtesy Caroline Baumal, MD.)

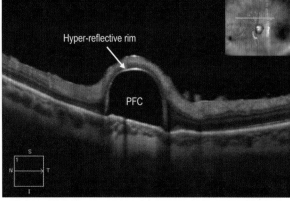

Figure 11.5.2 OCT through the subretinal perfluorocarbon liquid (PFC) liquid droplet (corresponding to Figure 11.5.1) shows a completely hyporeflective space occupied by the PFC. There is a distinct rim of hyper-reflectivity. The overlying retina is very thin because of a mechanical effect of the dense liquid. (Courtesy Caroline Baumal, MD.)

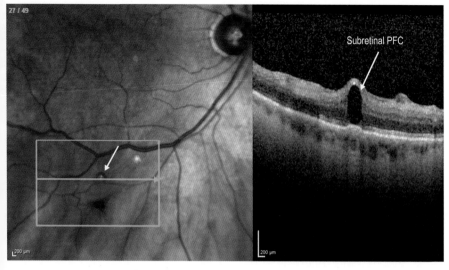

Figure 11.5.3 OCT through a small, retained subretinal PFC liquid droplet (arrows). The PFC appears to be within the retina although it is actually underneath the retina. (Courtesy Jeffrey S. Heier, MD.)

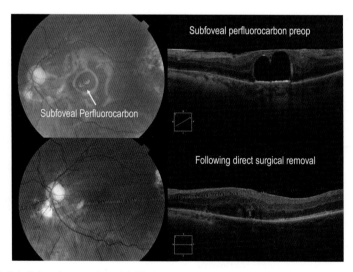

Figure 11.5.4 Color photograph and OCT show subfoveal PFC with silicone oil tamponade (top) and the same eye after surgical removal of the majority of the PFC via direct retinotomy (bottom).

Introduction: X-linked juvenile retinoschisis (XLRS) is the most common type of child-onset retinal degeneration in males and is caused by a mutation in the RS1 gene.

Clinical Features: There is almost always schisis in the fovea, which is often accompanied by schisis in the peripheral retina (50% of affected eyes), usually inferotemporally. The foveal schisis leads to a characteristic clinical appearance similar to cystoid macular edema with a radial spoke-like pattern (Figs. 11.6.1 and 11.6.2).

OCT Features: There is diffuse **splitting within multiple retinal layers** involving both the **inner** and **outer** retina. Within the macula, the **inner nuclear layer** is the most commonly affected layer (Fig. 11.6.3). However, the outer nuclear layer, ganglion cell layer, and nerve fiber layer can all be affected (Fig. 11.6.4). Unlike with typical cystoid macular edema (CME), the splitting in schisis can occur well outside the foveal area. Schisis may involve the peripheral retina, where OCT can be just as useful in confirming the diagnosis (Fig. 11.6.5)

Ancillary Testing: Fluorescein angiography (FA) can be helpful in distinguishing this condition from CME caused by other diseases. In XLRS, there is no macular leakage on FA. Electroretinography (ERG) testing shows a negative waveform. Genetic testing is confirmatory.

Treatment: There is no specific treatment for the disease, but treatment of retinal complications such as retinal detachment may be required.

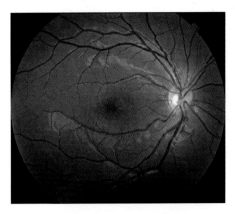

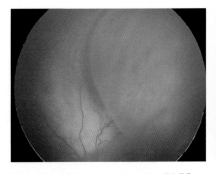

Figure 11.6.2 Color photograph of XLRS shows bullous peripheral schisis, which is most commonly located inferotemporally.

Figure 11.6.1 Color photograph of X-linked juvenile retinoschisis (XLRS) shows cystoid changes within the fovea arranged in a characteristic radial spoke-like pattern.

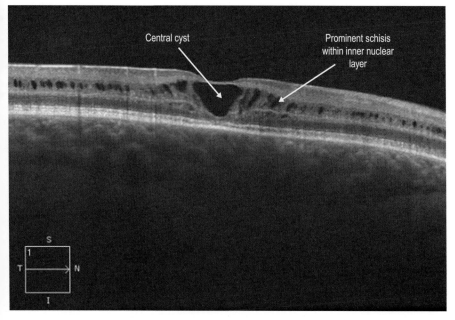

Figure 11.6.3 OCT of XLRS shows prominent schisis mostly within the inner nuclear layer. There is a central cyst present.

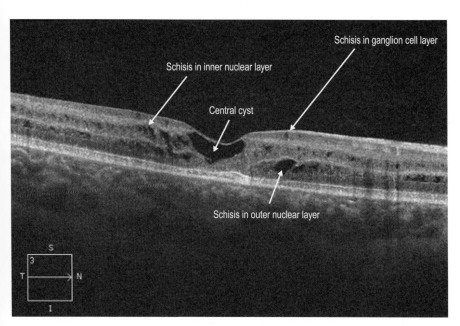

Figure 11.6.4 OCT of XLRS (corresponding to Figure 11.6.1) shows schisis within the ganglion cell layer, inner nuclear layer, and outer nuclear layer. There is also a central cyst present.

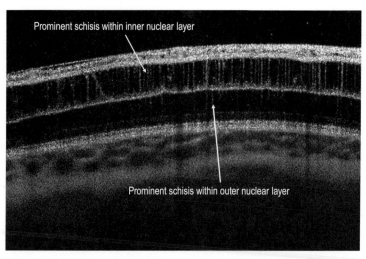

Figure 11.6.5 Peripheral OCT of XLRS (corresponding to Figure 11.6.2) shows peripheral schisis with extensive splitting of the inner and outer nuclear layers.

PART 4: Vaso-Occlusive Disorders

Section 12: Diabetic Retinopathy 120

12.1 *Non-Proliferative Diabetic Retinopathy* 120
Omar Abu-Qamar

12.2 *Non-Proliferative Diabetic Retinopathy With Macular Edema* 126
Omar Abu-Qamar

12.3 *Proliferative Diabetic Retinopathy* 130
Omar Abu-Qamar

Section 13: Retinal Vein Obstruction 136

13.1 *Branch Retinal Vein Obstruction* 136
Eugenia Custo Greig

13.2 *Central Retinal Vein Obstruction* 140
Eugenia Custo Greig

Section 14: Retinal Artery Obstruction 144

14.1 *Branch Retinal Artery Obstruction* 144
14.2 *Central Retinal Artery Obstruction* 148
14.3 *Cilioretinal Artery Obstruction* 152
14.4 *Paracentral Acute Middle Maculopathy* 154

Introduction: In 2019, 463 million adults were estimated to be living with diabetes. Around 35% of patients with diabetes suffer from diabetic retinopathy (DR) and 12% suffer from vision threatening DR. Therefore, DR remains the most common cause of new-onset blindness in people between the ages of 20 and 74 years in developed countries. The prevalence and severity of DR are affected by the duration of diabetes, glycemic control, and the presence of concurrent hypertension.

Clinical Features: In the early stages, non-proliferative diabetic retinopathy (NPDR) is typically asymptomatic. Retinal manifestations of DR are caused by a microangiopathy that manifests itself as microaneurysms (MA); the hallmarks of NPDR are intraretinal hemorrhage, cotton wool spots, hard exudates, and, in some eyes, macular edema (Fig. 12.1.1). Venous beading and intraretinal microvascular abnormalities (IRMA) may happen in severe NPDR. NPDR is subclassified as mild, moderate, or severe based on the presence and extent of these findings.

OCT Features: Although OCT scanning is not needed for the diagnosis of any form of DR, OCT findings of DR are well characterized on OCT. However, small intraretinal hemorrhages seen in the early stages of diabetes may not be detectable on even high-resolution line scans. MAs appear as **hyper-reflective foci**, mostly within the outer half of the retina, usually spanning more than one retinal layer. They typically have an **inner homogenous lumen** with moderate reflectivity surrounded by a **hyper-reflective rim** (sometimes referred to as the ring sign). Hyporeflectivity around the microaneurysm is usually associated with leakage on fluorescein angiography. Microaneurysm closure may be associated with resolution of hyper-reflectivity or by a smaller lumen with heterogenous hyper-reflectivity (Figs. 12.1.2 to 12.1.4).

Cotton wool spots appear as areas of moderate hyper-reflectivity within the nerve fiber layer. Larger cotton wool spots show shadowing. Hard exudates are also seen as small, relatively well-demarcated hyper-reflective clusters usually deeper within the retina and may span multiple layers. Another OCT parameter seen in diabetic patients is presence of hyper-reflective foci within the outer retina on OCT scanning, especially in diabetic macular edema (Fig. 12.1.2). These hyper-reflective foci probably represent a variety of microstructural pathologies including microaneurysms and hard exudates. The baseline amount of hyper-reflective foci seems to correlate positively with HbA1c values.

Diabetic macular edema (DME) is the primary cause of visual loss in NPDR and is covered in Chapter 12.2.

OCTA Features: Clinical features of NPDR detectable on OCTA include microaneurysms, intraretinal microvascular abnormalities (IRMA), capillary dropout, pruning of vessels, and enlargement of the foveal avascular zone (Figs. 12.1.5 and 12.1.6). Similar to fluorescein angiography (FA), MAs appear as small dilations of capillaries on en face OCTA images. However, up to 50% of MAs visible on FA are not visible on OCTA. This can be attributed to the slower (or absent) flow inside the MA below the OCTA signal detection threshold. IRMA appear as irregular, dilated, or looped capillaries within the retinal plane (Fig. 12.1.6).

Unlike FA, OCTA enables visualization of the various retinal capillary plexuses in isolation, which may be important in evaluating for ischemia. Furthermore, OCTA can be more precise in evaluating areas of ischemia and leakage because of the lack of obscuring fluorescein dye.

Various approaches have been implemented to quantify changes on OCTA images. Vascular density metric, for example, can indicate diabetic vascular changes prior to clinically detectable DR. Such metrics have the potential to be used as objective clinical end points.

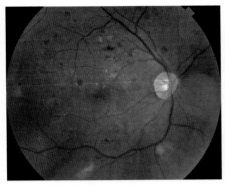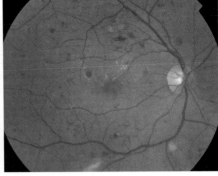

Figure 12.1.1 Color fundus photograph showing intraretinal hemorrhages, microaneurysms, cotton wool spots, and hard exudates in a patient with NPDR. The red-free photo is especially useful in evaluating for microaneurysms.

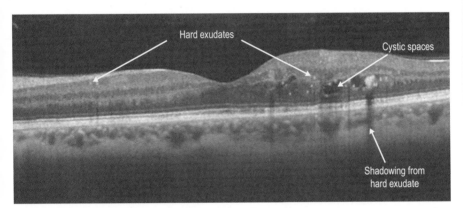

Figure 12.1.2 OCT line scan in a diabetic shows hyper-reflective clusters most likely representing hard exudates between the outer plexiform and the outer nuclear layer.

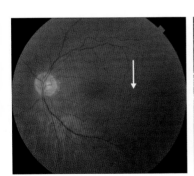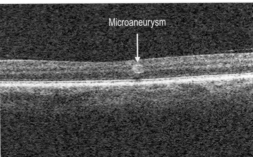

Figure 12.1.3 Photo and OCT line scan through a microaneurysm (white line) showing a discrete, well-demarcated area of hyper-reflectivity characteristic of diabetic microaneurysms.

Ancillary Testing: FA in NPDR is invaluable in looking for microaneurysms, areas of macular and peripheral ischemia, and neovascularization. Red-free photographs may enhance visualization of the microaneurysms. Ultra-wide-field FA can detect areas of ischemia and neovascularization not seen on 7-field FA imaging.

Treatment: Glycemic control and management of co-morbidities such as blood lipid levels and hypertension are the mainstays of NPDR management. Anti-vascular endothelial growth factor agents used in severe NPDR can cause regression in severity of the NPDR.

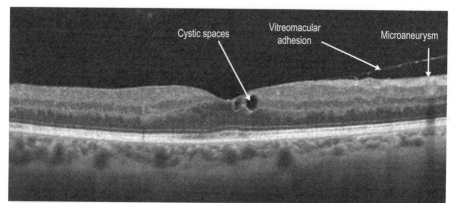

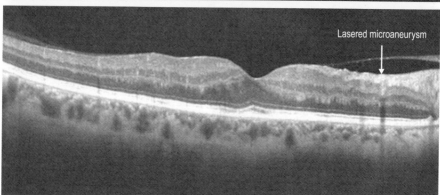

Figure 12.1.4 The upper image is a line scan through a microaneurysm showing an inner retinal discrete microaneurysm spanning several layers with a hyper-reflective border and relatively hypo-reflective lumen (arrow). The bottom image shows a post-focal laser OCT line scan through the same microaneurysm showing shrinkage and hyper-reflectivity throughout the now occluded lumen.

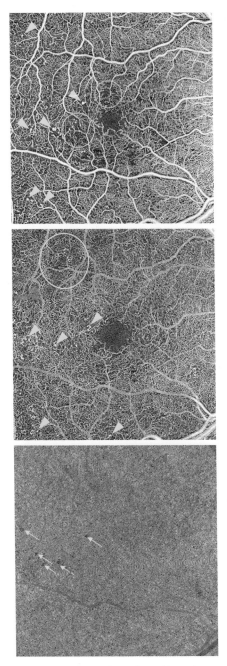

Figure 12.1.5 OCTA 6 × 6 mm *en face* image of a patient with moderate non-proliferative diabetic retinopathy (NPDR). The superficial capillary plexus, deep capillary plexus, and choriocapillaris slabs are shown in the upper, middle, and lower images, respectively. Diabetic vascular changes are demonstrated, such as foveal avascular zone irregularity, microaneurysms (arrowheads), capillary dropout (circled), and choriocapillaris flow voids, a newly described OCTA finding (arrows).

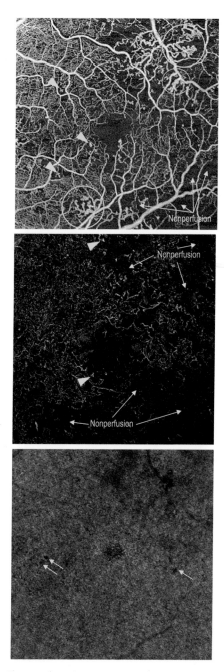

Figure 12.1.6 OCTA 6 × 6 mm *en face* of a patient with severe non-proliferative diabetic retinopathy (NPDR). The superficial capillary plexus, deep capillary plexus, and choriocapillaris slabs are shown in the upper, middle, and lower images, respectively. More severe diabetic vascular changes can be appreciated in this case (especially temporally). In addition to microaneurysms (arrowheads), large areas of capillary dropout and choriocapillaris flow voids (arrows), notice the intraretinal microvascular abnormalities (IRMA), which appear as pruned and dilated vessels/loops (circled).

| # Non-Proliferative Diabetic Retinopathy With Macular Edema

Introduction: Diabetic retinopathy is estimated to affect one-third of people with diabetes. The prevalence and severity are affected by the duration of diabetes, glycemic control, and the presence of concurrent hypertension. Diabetic macular edema (DME) can affect up to 7% of patients with diabetes and is the most common cause of moderate visual loss in diabetic patients. It can occur at any level of diabetic retinopathy.

Clinical Features: The hallmark of DME is retinal thickening in the posterior pole, and the classic clinical descriptions of DME includes focal, diffuse, and cystoid (CME), based on the clinical and angiographic appearance (Fig. 12.2.1). Focal macular edema is characterized by focal leaking microaneurysms giving a well-circumscribed area of thickening often associated with hard exudates. DME is characterized by more widespread vascular abnormalities giving larger areas of thickening, a paucity of hard exudates, and cystic changes in the retina. CME associated with DME appears similar to CME from other causes. It is not unusual for affected eyes to manifest two or all three of these subtypes.

OCT Features (Figs 12.2.2 to 12.2.4): In clinical practice as well as in studies, OCT is being used on a routine basis in the diagnosis of DME. Moreover, it is the single most important ancillary test in the management of DME. It is helpful for confirming the clinical diagnosis, choosing the initial therapy, and monitoring the edema on follow-up or after treatment. Quantitative changes in the OCT in DME are important in following the progression as well as the response to therapy. The mean **central subfield thickness** in the macular map is most often used. More than the absolute number, however, following the evolution of the thickness as well as the spread of the area of thickness is important in the evaluation and follow-up of DME.

The OCT appearance of DME can be categorized into four major types:

▸ Thickening of the fovea with **homogenous optical reflectivity** throughout the whole layer of the retina.

▸ Thickening of the fovea with markedly **decreased optical reflectivity** in mostly the outer retinal layers (cystoid changes).

▸ Thickening of the fovea with **subfoveal fluid** accumulation and distinct outer border of **detached retina**.

▸ Thickening of the fovea with **epiretinal membrane** formation with or without apparent **vitreofoveal traction**.

The qualitative assessment of OCT scans in DME are proving increasingly important in predicting outcome as well as determining which patients will respond best to individualized treatment. Moreover, OCT may also show foveal microstructural changes such as **disruption of the IS–OS/ ellipsoid layer and of the external limiting membrane**, which may be correlated to visual acuity in DME. Presence of **hyper-reflective foci** may also be associated with severity of the edema in DME and may reduce significantly with successful treatment of edema. Ischemia of the retina may also be associated with disorganization of the retinal inner layers (DRIL).

OCTA Features: OCTA use in DME is limited by its inability to detect leakage. Nevertheless, OCTA images are intrinsically co-registered with structural OCT images, allowing evaluation of microvascular alterations such as ischemia and microaneurysms in relation to edema. This is especially advantageous in areas of leakage where the FA dye can obscure the view. Similar to other causes of exudative maculopathy, DME can appear as areas of hyper-reflectivity on *en face* OCTA images, a feature thought to be caused by suspended scattering particles in motion (SSPiM) (Fig. 12.2.5). SSPiM may resolve and leave behind hard exudate.

Ancillary Testing: Fluorescein angiography (FA) will show microaneurysms in the early and intermediate stages with leakage later on in DME. FA can also be used to evaluate for macular ischemia. Wide-field angiography can be used to evaluate for peripheral ischemia and retinal neovascularization.

Treatment: Treatment for DME includes anti-vascular endothelial growth factor therapy, focal or grid laser photocoagulation, intravitreal steroids, and vitrectomy surgery.

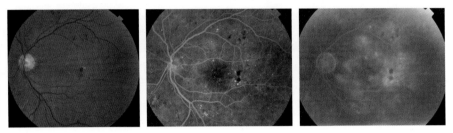

Figure 12.2.1 Fundus photograph of a diabetic patient shows numerous microaneurysms, hard exudates, and scattered cotton wool spots. Early frame fluorescein highlights the microaneurysms and late phase shows diffuse leakage at the macula.

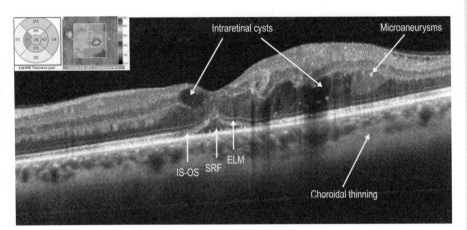

Figure 12.2.2 OCT scanning through the retina shows thickening with outer retinal cystic changes (arrows). The area and extent of thickening can be followed by the false color rendering of the thickness map over the C-scan (inset). The retinal thickness map also provides quantitative information about thickening and is useful in gauging effect of treatment. Note the hyper-reflective clusters in the outer retina, the trace subretinal fluid or SRF (arrow), and the relatively well-preserved external limiting membrane (arrow). The IS–OS/ellipsoid layer shows some disruption centrally (arrow).

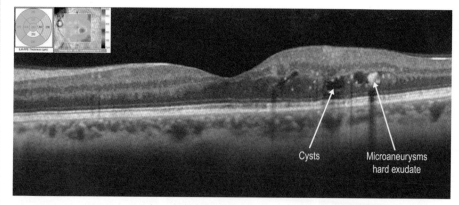

Figure 12.2.3 OCT scan of the same patient after focal laser therapy. The edema and cysts are reduced, as is the retinal thickness on the thickness map. Also, the normal architecture of the IS–OS ellipsoid layer seems relatively well restored.

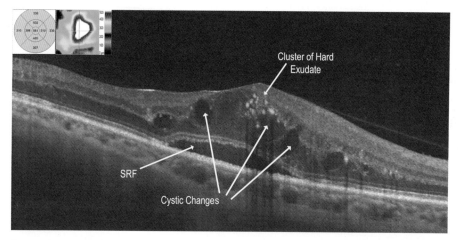

Figure 12.2.4 OCT scan through the fovea showing diffuse retinal thickening on false color rendering of the thickness map (inset). Cystic changes, subretinal fluid (SRF), and a cluster of hard exudate are also shown (arrows).

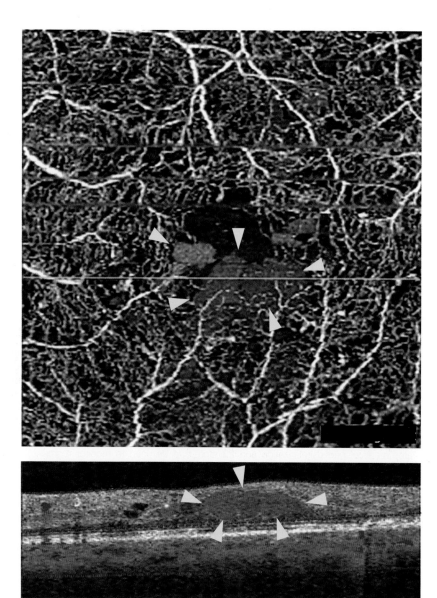

Figure 12.2.5 OCTA 3 × 3 mm *en face* image (top) and a structural OCT B-scan with flow overlay (bottom) in diabetic macular edema is shown. Note the area of hyper-reflectivity on the *en face* image (arrowheads), which corresponds to edema. The false flow signal is caused by suspended scattering particles in motion (SSPiM) present in the fluid.

12.3 | Proliferative Diabetic Retinopathy

Introduction: Proliferative diabetic retinopathy (PDR) is characterized by pathologic retinal neovascularization. It can arise from the optic disc (NVD), retina (elsewhere; NVE), and/or the iris (NVI).

Clinical Features: Retinal neovascularization is a hallmark of PDR, which can be seen at the slit lamp as fine networks of blood vessels extending from the retina into the vitreous cavity (Fig. 12.3.1). These vessels can cause visual loss secondary to vitreous hemorrhage and can induce preretinal fibrosis leading to tractional retinal detachment, retinoschisis, macular edema, and combined traction/rhegmatogenous retinal detachment (RD).

Neovascularization can occur at the disc or elsewhere in the retina. It may be preceded by intraretinal microvascular abnormalities (IRMA), which represent a severe form of NPDR.

OCT Features: The typical findings of NPDR are also seen in PDR. In addition, NVD and NVE may manifest as **loops of hyper-reflective blood vessels** projecting from the retina into the vitreous, either at the disc or elsewhere (Fig. 12.3.2). In contrast, areas of IRMA are seen as **disorganization** of the inner retinal vascular architecture with occasional projection beyond the internal limiting membrane, but with no disruption of the hyaloid face (Fig. 12.3.3). The hyaloid may be **thickened** in these cases. In some cases with NVD or NVE, **traction of the retina** with or without retinal detachment may be seen (Fig. 12.3.4).

OCTA Features: OCTA can show macular ischemia with enlargement of the foveal avascular zone and additional areas of ischemia. NVD and NVE are seen as loops of blood vessels that project into the vitreous cavity, in contrast to IRMA, which are contained within the retinal plane and respect the inner limiting membrane (Fig. 12.3.5).

OCTA can be used to quantify areas of neovascularization, which is useful because leakage may confound such quantification on fluorescein angiography (FA) (Fig. 12.3.6). OCTA clearly delineates areas of neovascularization and therefore can be used to monitor regression and regrowth (Fig. 12.3.7).

Ancillary Testing: FA, especially wide field, is the most useful ancillary test in diagnosing diabetic retinopathy. FA of the areas of neovascularization shows profuse dye leakage. Ischemic areas may also be delineated on the FA.

Treatment: PDR is treated with pan-retinal photocoagulation. As it has become clear that elevated levels of VEGF are a critical driver of neovascularization in PDR, increasingly, anti-VEGF therapy is being used as an adjunct in the treatment. There are reports that anti-VEGF injections may induce regression of PDR, but they can cause increased fibrosis of the regressing neovascularization possibly resulting in increased traction on the retina. Vitrectomy is the mainstay of therapy for non-clearing vitreous hemorrhage and traction-related complications of PDR, when pan-retinal photocoagulation fails or is not possible to perform.

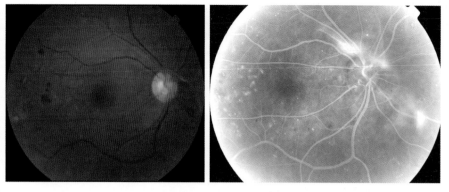

Figure 12.3.1 Neovascularization of the optic disc and of the retina is seen on the photograph and the accompanying fluorescein angiography.

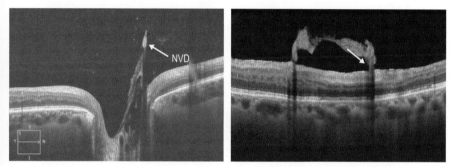

Figure 12.3.2 OCT section through the area of the neovascularization of the optic disc (NVD) reveals hyper-reflective neovascularization into the vitreous cavity (arrow). The adjacent picture shows a high-resolution OCT scan through an area of neovascularization of the retina.

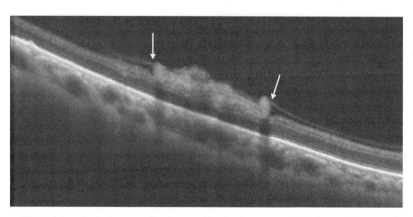

Figure 12.3.3 Intraretinal microvascular abnormalities/early neovascularization starting to project into the hyaloid cavity but with an intact, thickened posterior hyaloid face over it (arrows).

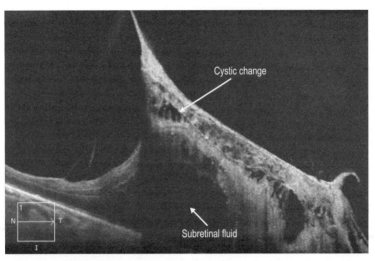

Figure 12.3.4 Tractional retinal detachment. There is thickened preretinal fibrosis and a tractional detachment.

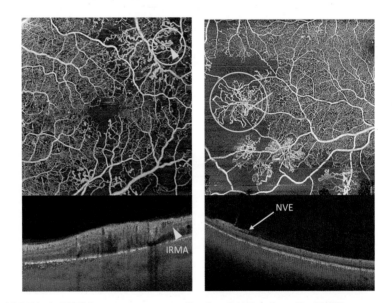

Figure 12.3.5 Left: OCTA from a severe non-proliferative diabetic retinopathy (NPDR) case demonstrating intraretinal microvascular abnormalities (arrowheads) and the corresponding OCT B-scan with flow overlay passing through the lesion demonstrating that the lesion is limited to the retinal plane. Right: OCTA from a PDR case demonstrating neovascularization of the retina (NVE; arrows). The vascular lesion breaches the internal limiting membrane and extends up to the posterior hyaloid as demonstrated on the corresponding B-scan with flow overlay.

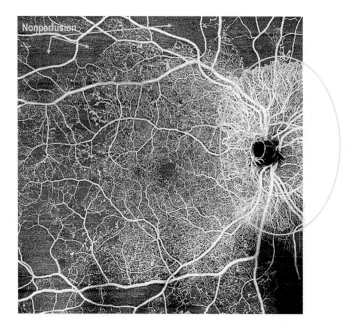

Figure 12.3.6 Wide-field 12 × 12 mm OCTA in proliferative diabetic retinopathy demonstrating large areas of ischemia more pronounced in the periphery (arrows) and neovascularization of the optic disc (circle).

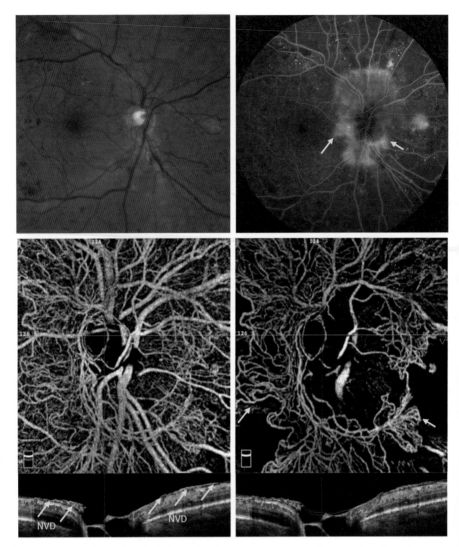

Figure 12.3.7 Color fundus photo (upper left) from the same proliferative diabetic retinopathy case shown in Fig. 12.3.6 cropped around the optic nerve head demonstrating neovascularization of the optic disc (NVD). Late-phase fluorescein angiography (upper right) showing leakage from the NVD at the optic nerve head. Note that the NVD details are obscured by the leaking dye. OCTA *en face* scan of the whole retina slab (lower left) and a custom slab (lower right) clearly delineates the NVD (arrows).

Branch Retinal Vein Obstruction

Branch retinal vein obstruction (BRVO) is characterized by hemorrhages, ischemia, and edema along the territory of the occluded vein, which can produce decreased vision and metamorphopsia.

Epidemiology: BRVO usually occurs in patients in their fifth or sixth decade of life. The prevalence of BRVO in the United States is estimated at just under 1%. There does not appear to be any racial or ethnic predilection. Hypertension is the most common risk factor and disease of the adjacent arterial wall secondary to diabetes, hypertension, or arteriosclerosis usually compresses the venous wall at a crossing point.

Clinical Features: Patients may complain of visual blurring, distortion, metamorphopsia, or floaters. On examination, there are intraretinal flame and blot-shaped hemorrhages along a retinal vein, which almost never cross the horizontal raphe (Fig. 13.1.1). Cotton wool spots, dilation, and tortuosity of the involved retinal vein, retinal edema in the area drained by the occluded branch, collateral vessels, and occasionally retinal neovascularization and vitreous hemorrhage may be seen. Vision loss is usually caused by retinal edema and may sometimes be secondary to retinal ischemia and neovascularization.

OCT Features: OCT shows retinal thickening and edema. Macular thickness scans will show retinal thickening, usually confined to half the macula. This may be especially prominent in the internal limiting membrane–retinal pigment epithelium (ILM-RPE) map. Line scans through the macula will show diffuse retinal edema and cystic (hyporeflective) spaces in the outer retina. Some subretinal fluid or a neurosensory retinal detachment may also be observed. Hard exudates may appear as small hyper-reflective intraretinal spots on the OCT. Macular thickness and ILM-RPE scans are particularly valuable in monitoring edema over time and the effects of treatment. (Figs. 13.1.2 and 13.1.3)

OCTA Features: OCTA shows capillary non-perfusion at each retinal plexus. The deep capillary plexus is the most affected vascular bed. Wide-field OCTA imaging can be used to assess extent of areas of retinal non-perfusion. Non-perfused areas identified on OCTA correlate closely with those found on FA (Fig. 13.1.4).

Microvascular changes such as foveal avascular zone enlargement, microaneurysms, telangiectasias, and collateral vessel formation can be seen (Fig. 13.1.5). Cross-section shows areas of intraretinal hemorrhage and cystoid spaces in the outer retina. Edema secondary to venous obstructions can lead to segmentation errors and slab segmentation should therefore be checked on B-scan prior to en face interpretation. OCTA can be used to confirm the presence of retinal or optic disc neovascularization.

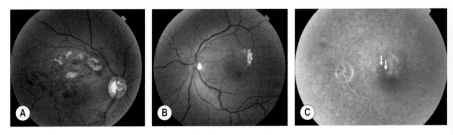

Figure 13.1.1 (A,B) Branch retinal vein obstruction with a range of findings. Note hemorrhages along the blocked blood vessels and the cottonwool spots (A) as well as the hard exudates (B). (C) A late frame fluorescein angiogram with collaterals (arrows) and leakage from the vessels.

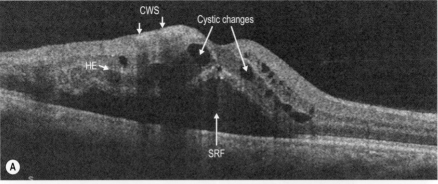

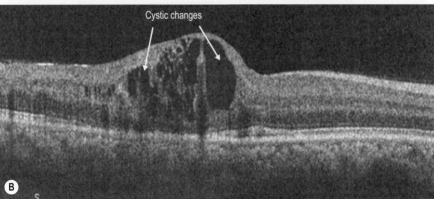

Figure 13.1.2 OCT scans through the macula of the patient (A), with diffuse retinal thickening and cystic changes (arrows). Note the cottonwool spots (CWS) (arrows) in the nerve fiber layer that cause shadowing of the layers beneath them. Some hard exudates (HE) are noted (arrow) as hyper-reflective clusters deeper within the retina and spanning several layers. Subretinal fluid (SRF) is also seen. (B) Note that only part of the retina is thickened unlike in central retinal vein obstruction.

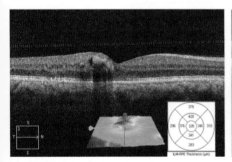
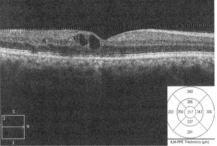

Figure 13.1.3 Shows OCT scans in the same patient after treatment with laser and anti-vascular endothelial growth factor therapy, with thinning of the retina seen on the line and macular thickness scans as well as a smaller geographic spread of the thickening seen on the internal limiting membrane–retinal pigment epithelium (ILM-RPE) overlay.

Ancillary Testing: Fluorescein angiography can be of value to assess perfusion. It may also be used to confirm neovascularization.

Treatment: Treatment of a branch retinal vein obstruction is a classic observation and is treated by focal grid laser if needed to the area with edema. Anti-vascular endothelial growth factor therapy is being used as an effective treatment against macular edema in BRVO. Scatter laser can be used to treat neovascularization.

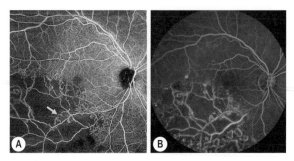

Figure 13.1.4 (A) 12 × 12 mm OCTA scan of the superficial retinal layer in a patient with branch retinal vein obstruction after laser therapy. Arrow points to collateral vessel formation. (B) Fluorescein angiography for the same patient. Area of non-perfusion is seen inferotemporally on both images.

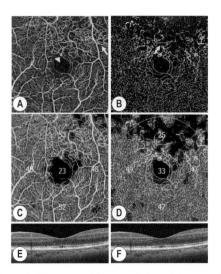

Figure 13.1.5 (A,B) 3 × 3 mm OCTA scans of the superficial and deep capillary plexus in a patient with branch retinal vein obstruction. Note parafoveal microaneurysm (arrowhead) in (A). Areas of neovascularization can be seen in both capillary plexuses (yellow arrows, A,B). Vessel density maps (C,D) show pronounced vascular loss in the deep capillary plexus. (E,F) Segmentation boundaries are shown for each image.

Central retinal vein obstruction (CRVO) is characterized by obstruction of the central retinal vein at or proximal to the lamina cribrosa resulting in unilateral, usually sudden painless vision loss secondary to macular edema and ischemia.

Epidemiology: The incidence of CRVO in the United States is 30,000 per annum. Risk factors include age > 55 years, a history of glaucoma, systemic hypertension, smoking, hyperlipidemia, diabetes, atherosclerosis, coagulopathies, vasculitis, and oral contraceptive use.

Clinical Features: Dilated, tortuous retinal veins and intraretinal hemorrhages are noted in all four quadrants (Fig. 13.2.1). Cottonwool spots, disc edema, and macular edema may also be seen. CRVO may be categorized as ischemic or non-ischemic. In ischemic CRVO, visual acuity tends to be worse (< 20/200), and there may be more cottonwool spots seen on examination. Non-ischemic CRVO is characterized by better visual acuity and the relative paucity of cotton-wool spots. Non-ischemic CRVO can convert to ischemic CRVO in about 20%–30% of cases. Although the diagnosis of CRVO can be made by the characteristic fundus appearance, perfusion and the presence of ischemia are best assessed by a fluorescein angiogram (FA).

OCT Features: Macular edema in CRVO is best evaluated by an OCT scan (Figs. 13.2.2 and 13.2.3). A line scan through the OCT shows diffuse thickening with hyporeflective spaces within the outer retinal layers consistent with cystoid macular edema. Some subretinal fluid may also be noted, which is most likely secondary to excess intraretinal fluid overflowing into the subretinal space.

A cube scan shows diffuse thickening. Central subfield thickness on a cube scan and the topography of the edema on the internal limiting membrane–retinal pigment epithelium (ILM-RPE) map are effective ways of identifying macular edema over serial visits and response to treatment and this correlates well to visual acuity in non-ischemic CRVO.

OCTA Features: OCTA identifies changes at each retinal plexus that would normally be obscured by dye leakage in FA (Fig. 13.2.4). It shows areas of non-perfusion affecting the superficial and deep vascular beds, as well as the choriocapillaris. As in branch retinal vein obstruction, the deep capillary plexus is most affected.

Microvascular changes in the superficial and deep retinal plexuses include collateral vessel formation, telangiectasias, and vascular thickening. At the superficial capillary plexus, parafoveal vessels appear tortuous and thinned. Enlarged foveal avascular zone after a CRVO is seen on OCTA and correlates with worse visual acuity outcomes (Fig. 13.2.5A,B).

In patients with ongoing macular edema, en face images are prone to segmentation artifact and should be interpreted in the context of the corresponding B-scan (Fig. 13.2.5C,D).

Ancillary Testing: Intravenous FA may show areas of blocked fluorescence from the intraretinal blood, staining of the vessel walls, a delayed arteriovenous phase, non-perfused areas, and perifoveal leakage. In the early stages, the presence of hemorrhage may block fluorescence and make it difficult to assess for ischemia. Moreover, the FA may not show the full extent of perifoveal leakage because of a lack of intact perifoveal vessels. Neovascularization of the retina in CRVO will show diffuse leakage from abnormal blood vessels.

Treatment: There is no known effective mechanism to treat macular ischemia in CRVO. However, macular edema may effectively be treated with intravitreal anti-vascular endothelial growth factor (VEGF) agents such as bevacizumab, ranibizumab, and aflibercept, as well as intravitreal corticosteroids. Neovascularization in CRVO is treated with pan retinal photocoagulation. Anti-VEGF agents may also be used as adjuncts in the treatment of neovascularization secondary to CRVO.

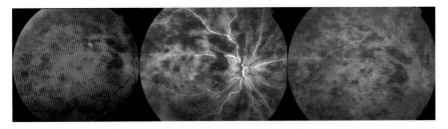

Figure 13.2.1 Fundus photo of an eye with central retinal vein obstruction shows four quadrants of intraretinal hemorrhages, cottonwool spots, and retinal edema. The fluorescein angiogram highlights the dilated, tortuous vessels. There is blockage because of the intraretinal hemorrhages.

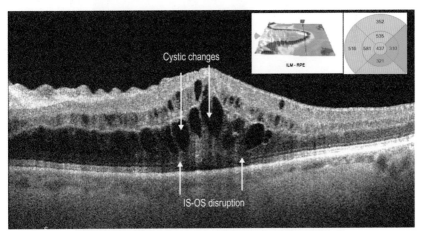

Figure 13.2.2 Intraretinal thickening is noted. Cystic changes are seen in the outer retina that span multiple retinal layers. There is some subretinal fluid. The thickening does not respect the horizontal raphe as seen on the thickness map (inset). There is ellipsoid IS-OS disruption seen (between bottom two white arrows).

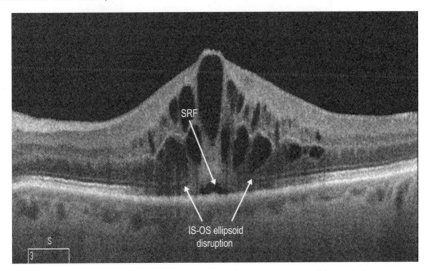

Figure 13.2.3 The same patient after treatment with anti-vascular endothelial growth factor agent. Note that the area of thickening has decreased. There is ellipsoid IS-OS disruption and subretinal fluid.

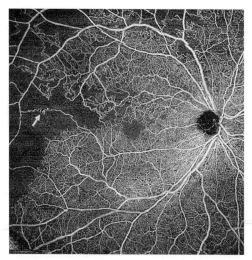

Figure 13.2.4 Superficial retina scan (12 × 12 mm) of a patient with CRVO after anti-vascular endothelial growth factor therapy. Non-perfused area can be seen superiorly and temporal to the fovea. Note collateral vessel formation (yellow arrow).

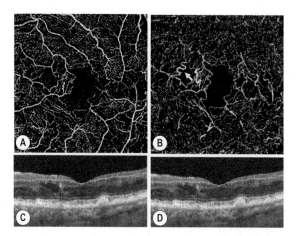

Figure 13.2.5 Macular OCTA scans (3 × 3 mm) of a patient with central retinal vein obstruction. (A) Superficial retinal layer. (B) The deep retinal layer. Note irregular, large foveal avascular zone in both images. Yellow arrow points to area of neovascularization in the deep retinal layer with vascular thickening. (C,D) B-scans through the macula with corresponding segmentation lines. Note cystic edema.

Introduction: The incidence of branch retinal artery obstruction (BRAO) is slightly less than that of central retinal artery obstruction (CRAO). Patients typically present with acute painless, monocular vision loss affecting a sector of the visual field. The most common etiology is an identifiable embolus, present in about two-thirds of cases.

Clinical Features: There is retinal whitening along the sector of retina supplied by the affected arterial branch from the central retinal artery (Fig. 14.1.1). The temporal hemisphere is most commonly affected. A visible embolus at the site of blockage, typically at a bifurcation point, is often apparent.

OCT Features: In the acute setting, there is **intense hyper-reflectivity of the inner retinal layers**, similar to that seen in CRAO (see Chapter 14.2) but limited to the sector of retina involved. Vertical, instead of horizontal, OCT cuts can help to make this distinction (Fig. 14.1.2). With time, the edema resolves, leaving attenuation and atrophy of the inner retinal layers, which can appear as thinning or even schisis-like changes (Fig. 14.1.3). OCTA allows isolated segmentation and visualization of the inner retinal vasculature, which can identify impaired vascular flow in the distribution of the affected branch retinal artery (Fig. 14.1.4).

Ancillary Testing: Fluorescein angiography can help in securing the diagnosis by revealing a sectoral perfusion deficiency in the acute setting (Fig. 14.1.5).

Treatment: No consistent treatment has demonstrated proven efficacy. Successful YAG laser embolectomy has been described in a few case reports.

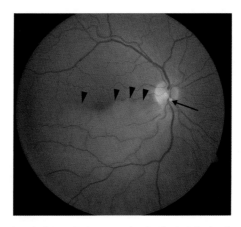

Figure 14.1.1 Color fundus photograph shows sectoral retinal whitening (arrowheads) in the distribution of the occluded branch retinal artery. There is also a visible embolus (arrow).

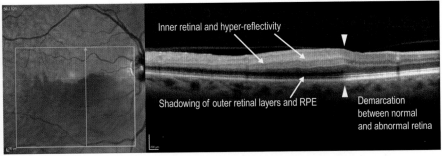

Inner retinal and hyper-reflectivity

Shadowing of outer retinal layers and RPE

Demarcation between normal and abnormal retina

Figure 14.1.2 OCT vertical cut shows inner retinal hyper-reflectivity and thickening only in the sectoral area of retina that is affected by the acute branch retinal artery obstruction (BRAO) (left of arrowheads). As with the case in central retinal artery obstruction (CRAO), the inner hyper-reflectivity in the affected region causes shadowing of the outer layers, which attenuates the signal from the outer retina and retinal pigment epithelium (RPE).

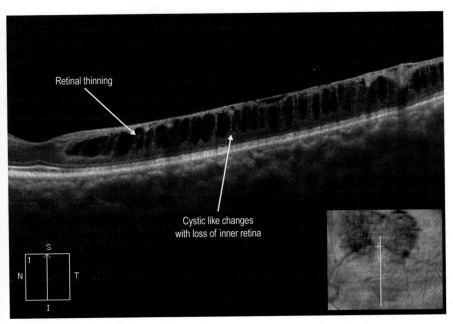

Retinal thinning

Cystic like changes with loss of inner retina

Figure 14.1.3 OCT vertical scan of an old BRAO, which occurred 7 years prior, shows inner retinal atrophy with schisis-like changes in the affected superior macula.

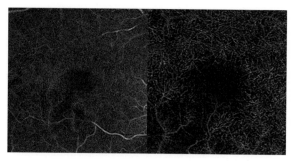

Figure 14.1.4 OCTA *en face* images (6 × 6, left; 3 × 3, right) in the setting of a subacute inferotemporal BRAO show impairment of retinal vascular flow in the distribution of the involved branch retinal artery.

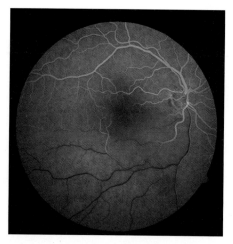

Figure 14.1.5 Fluorescein angiography (corresponding to Figure 14.1.1) shows a significant perfusion delay in the sector of retina affected by the branch retinal artery obstruction.

Introduction: Central retinal artery obstruction has an incidence of approximately 1 in 10,000 and typically occurs in the seventh decade, affecting men more frequently than woman. Patients present with sudden, profound, painless, monocular vision loss.

Clinical Features: The classic finding is retinal whitening with a central cherry-red spot in the acute setting (Fig. 14.2.1). This corresponds to edema of the inner retina, which is most pronounced in the macula due to the prominent nerve fiber and ganglion cell layer in this location. The central fovea, however, lacks inner retinal layers and, therefore, the underlying retinal pigment epithelium (RPE) and choroidal pigment show through, giving the cherry-red spot.

OCT Features: In the **acute** setting, there is **intense hyper-reflectivity of the inner retinal layers** (Fig. 14.2.2), corresponding to edema of the retinal layers supplied by the inner retinal vascular supply from the central retinal artery (watershed zone is between inner nuclear and outer plexiform layers). This hyper-reflectivity creates a **shadowing effect, which degrades the normal signal from the outer retinal layers**, exaggerating contrast between them. **Later**, the edema resolves leaving **attenuation and atrophy** of the inner retinal layers (Fig. 14.2.3). OCTA allows isolated segmentation and visualization of the inner retinal vasculature, which can aid in the diagnosis of central retinal artery obstruction (CRAO) (Figs. 14.2.4 and 14.2.5). In some cases, OCTA can also help differentiate CRAO from ophthalmic artery obstruction by visualizing the presence (or absence) of perfused posterior ciliary arteries (Fig. 14.2.4).

Ancillary Testing: Fluorescein angiography is helpful in assessing the perfusion status of the retina and can confirm the diagnosis of CRAO in the acute or subacute setting (Fig. 14.2.6) when suspected on clinical grounds.

Treatment: Although numerous therapies have been attempted, with occasional case reports documenting improvement, none have proven clinical efficacy compared with the natural history.

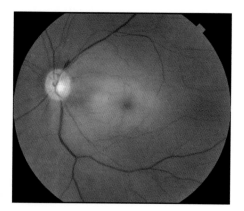

Figure 14.2.1 Color fundus photograph shows a classic cherry-red spot in acute central retinal artery obstruction (CRAO). There is also a superior optic disc hemorrhage.

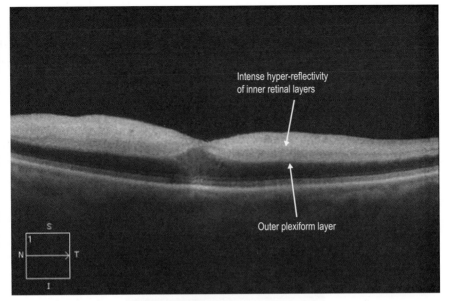

Intense hyper-reflectivity
of inner retinal layers

Outer plexiform layer

Figure 14.2.2 OCT (corresponding to Fig. 14.2.1) shows fairly homogeneous hyper-reflectivity and thickening of the inner retinal layers with a sharp demarcation at the level of the outer plexiform layer. The hyporeflectivity of the outer retinal layers is exaggerated by a shadowing effect caused by the overlying edema.

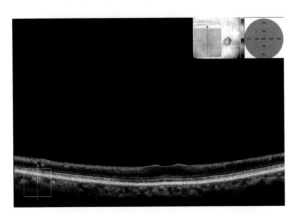

Figure 14.2.3 OCT 4 months after acute CRAO shows diffuse thinning of the inner retina.

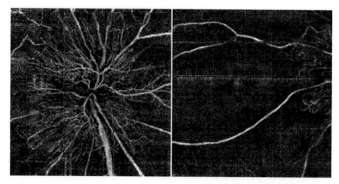

Figure 14.2.4 OCTA *en face* image of the inner retina shows profound impairment of global retinal artery perfusion due to acute CRAO (right). The optic nerve head vessels remain perfused (left) because these vessels are supplied by the posterior ciliary arteries, which are patent in this case but could be impaired in the setting of an ophthalmic artery obstruction.

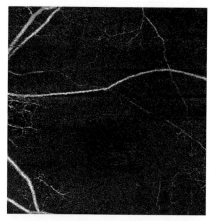

Figure 14.2.5 OCTA *en face* image of subacute CRAO shows profound impairment in arterial perfusion, although there are some areas of reperfusion present.

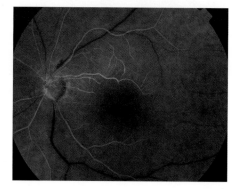

Figure 14.2.6 Fluorescein angiography in the subacute setting of a CRAO at 34 seconds shows a global, severe delay in filling time of both the arterial and venous circulation. There is also severe central macular ischemia.

Cilioretinal Artery Obstruction

Introduction: Cilioretinal artery obstruction (CiRAO) represents the rarest type of retinal vascular disease accounting for less than 10% of retinal arterial obstructions. A cilioretinal artery is only present in 20–30% of individuals. CiRAO can occur isolated, in conjunction with a central retinal vein obstruction (CRVO), or associated with arteritic ischemic optic neuropathy from giant cell arteritis. Patients typically report an acute, painless central scotoma or decrease in central visual acuity. When isolated or associated with CRVO, they have a generally good prognosis for at least partial visual recovery.

Clinical Features: There is localized retinal whitening due to inner retinal edema corresponding to the distribution of the cilioretinal artery (Fig. 14.3.1).

OCT Features: **Localized inner retinal hyper-reflectivity**, similar to that seen in branch retinal artery obstruction but localized to the distribution of the cilioretinal artery, is seen acutely (Fig. 14.3.2). Later, OCT will show thinning of the retina in the region supplied by the cilioretinal artery, which is best appreciated by a retinal thickness segmentation map (Fig. 14.3.3).

Ancillary Testing: Fluorescein angiography in the acute setting is helpful to confirm the diagnosis. The cilioretinal artery normally fills with the choroidal circulation a second or two earlier than the retinal circulation, a key distinguishing factor from central or branch retinal artery obstructions.

Treatment: No treatment is of proven clinical efficacy. Corticosteroids are indicated to prevent further visual loss in the setting of giant cell arteritis but rarely improve vision.

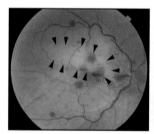

Figure 14.3.1 Color fundus photograph shows localized retinal whitening in the superior macula (arrowheads) corresponding to the distribution of the cilioretinal artery. There are also intraretinal hemorrhages, disc edema, and dilated and tortuous veins due to concomitant central retinal vein obstruction (CRVO).

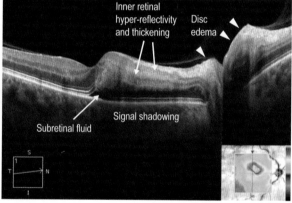

Inner retinal hyper-reflectivity and thickening Disc edema

Signal shadowing

Subretinal fluid

Figure 14.3.2 OCT (corresponding to Figure 14.3.1) in the acute setting of a cilioretinal artery obstruction (CiRAO) shows retinal hyper-reflectivity and thickening of the inner retinal layers with underlying shadowing. There is also associated subretinal fluid and disc edema (arrowheads) resulting from concomitant central retinal vein obstruction (CRVO).

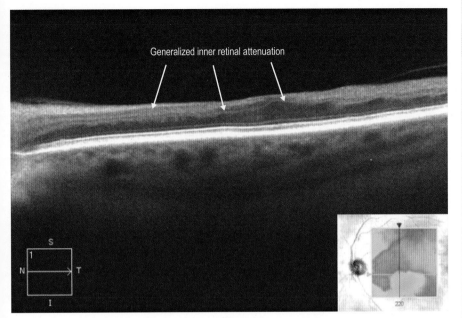

Generalized inner retinal attenuation

Figure 14.3.3 OCT many years after a cilioretinal artery obstruction shows generalized inner retinal attenuation. Corresponding retinal thickness segmentation map (inset) shows retinal thinning in a region corresponding to the area supplied by the cilioretinal artery.

| ## Paracentral Acute Middle Maculopathy

Introduction: Paracentral acute middle maculopathy (PAMM) represents a distinct clinical finding whereby the middle retinal layers in the macula are focally injured due to acute vascular insufficiency, which is best appreciated on OCT. PAMM can occur in isolation or in association with various retinal vascular disorders.

Clinical Features: Patients typically present with the subjective complaint of one or many paracentral scotomas. The clinical appearance of PAMM can be quite subtle and sometimes not apparent via ophthalmoscopy. If visible, there are distinct grayish, wedge-shaped lesions in a parafoveal configuration. Localized ischemia of the intermediate portion of the deep capillary plexus within the retinal vasculature is thought to be pathogenic. This is in distinction to localized ischemia of the superficial capillary plexus, which can manifest as a cottonwool spot. There is an association of PAMM with a number of retinal vascular disorders such as venous obstructions, arterial obstructions, diabetic retinopathy, and Purtscher retinopathy.

OCT Features: In the **acute phase** of PAMM, there is a **hyper-reflective band** (or bands) in the **middle retinal layers** at the confluence of the outer plexiform layer (OPL) and inner nuclear layer (INL), extending into the INL with underlying shadowing of the outer retina (Fig. 14.4.1). In the **chronic phase**, the hyper-reflectivity of the OPL and INL resolve and both become **atrophic** (Fig. 14.4.2). Separately, the deeper Henle fiber layer typically becomes hyporeflective. Of note, there is no disruption or involvement of the outer retina and IS/OS layer. The OCT features of PAMM are distinct from that of a cottonwool spot, where there is hyper-reflectivity and thickening of the inner macular layers, including the ganglion cell layer (GCL) and nerve fiber layer (NFL) (Fig. 14.4.3). To understand better the pathophysiology of PAMM, OCTA provides the unique ability to evaluate and study various planar segments of the retinal vasculature. Theoretically, this could elucidate pathologically impaired blood flow at the level of the intermediate and/or deep capillary plexuses. However, this feature has not yet been definitely identified in cases of PAMM. Such absence of abnormal flow in the deeper capillary plexuses on OCTA could be a result of the nature of the perfusion defect being momentary or a lack of adequate resolution from current OCTA technology.

Ancillary Testing: Near-infrared reflectance (NIR) images are helpful to visualize characteristic greyish (hyporeflective), paracentral, wedge-shaped defects. Color photography and fluorescein angiography are less helpful because they may appear normal. OCT is required to confirm the diagnosis of PAMM.

Treatment: There is no proven treatment. However, evaluation of patients with PAMM should be directed at uncovering a retinal vascular disorder or systemic disease that may be causative. Persistence of paracentral scotomas are common but may abate over time.

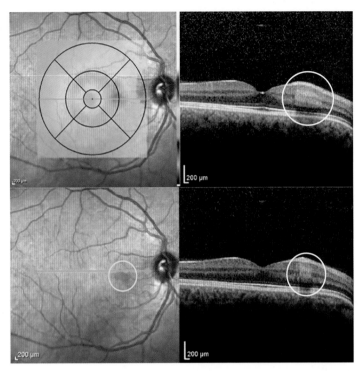

Figure 14.4.1 OCT in the acute phase of paracentral acute middle maculopathy (PAMM) (right side) shows hyper-reflectivity in a band- or plaque-like configuration involving the outer plexiform and inner nuclear layers (white circles). There is shadowing of the unaffected, underlying structures, including the IS/OS region. Near infrared reflectance image (bottom left) illustrates a gray, wedge-shaped irregularity (yellow circle), which corresponds to the abnormal defect on OCT. (Images courtesy Robin A. Vora, MD and Matthew Bedell, MD.)

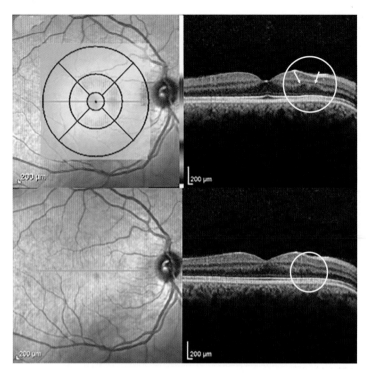

Figure 14.4.2 OCT 5 months after presentation (corresponding to Figure 14.4.1) shows the chronic features of PAMM. There is atrophy of the outer plexiform and inner nuclear layers focally in the area of the PAMM lesion (circles) along with focal hyporeflectivity of the Henle fiber layer (arrows). The outer retina and IS/OS region remain intact. Of note, the near infrared reflectance image appearance has normalized (bottom left). (Images courtesy Robin A. Vora, MD and Matthew Bedell, MD.)

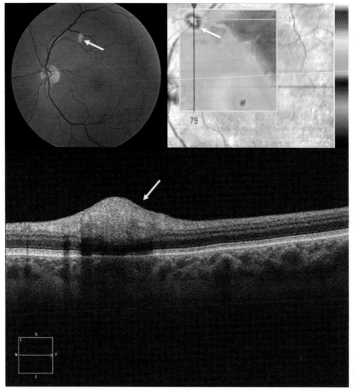

Figure 14.4.3 Color photograph and OCT of a cottonwool spot (arrows). OCT shows hyper-reflectivity and thickening of only the inner retina, specifically the nerve fiber layer and the ganglion cell layer. There is shadowing with reduced signal below the affected layers.

PART 5: Inherited Retinal Degenerations

Section 15: Inherited Retinal Degenerations 160

    15.1 Retinitis Pigmentosa 160
    15.2 Stargardt Disease 162
    15.3 Best Disease 164
    15.4 Cone Dystrophy 166

15.1 Retinitis Pigmentosa

Introduction: Retinitis pigmentosa (RP) encompasses a heterogeneous group of inherited disorders that result in loss of retinal cell function (starting with photoreceptors), preferentially in the peripheral retina. Eventually, the macula can be involved in late stages. The prevalence is approximately 1 in 5000. RP can be categorized several different ways: phenotype, cone–rod versus rod–cone dystrophies, via the inheritance patterns, or by the actual genetic defect, if it is known.

Clinical Features: Nyctalopia is a hallmark feature of the disease, which develops insidiously. Peripheral vision is impaired early, especially in rod–cone dystrophies, and is slowly progressive. Central vision can also be lost but typically occurs later in the disease course, although central vision can also be impaired at any point by secondary cystoid macular edema. Examination findings include characteristic bone spicule intraretinal deposits, vascular attenuation, and optic nerve pallor (Fig. 15.1.1).

OCT Features: In advanced RP cases, OCT demonstrates marked **attenuation of all retinal layers**, particularly of the **outer retina and photoreceptors** (Fig. 15.1.2). Milder or earlier forms of RP can show more subtle outer retinal atrophy adjacent to a **normal central macula** (Figs. 15.1.3 and 15.1.4). OCT can also be helpful to detect the presence of **cystoid macular edema** (Fig. 15.1.5), which is commonly associated with RP.

Ancillary Testing: Electrophysiologic testing, such as multifocal electroretinograms, are helpful to aid in the diagnosis of RP, especially in early cases where clinical findings are mild.

Treatment: There is no widely applicable treatment, but retinal prosthetic implants are now available for very advanced forms of RP.

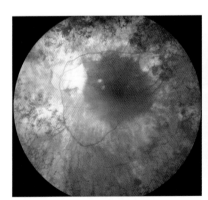

Figure 15.1.1 Color photograph of advanced retinitis pigmentosa shows peripheral bone spicule deposition encroaching into the macula, vascular attenuation, and optic nerve pallor. There is a central island of intact retinal pigment epithelium (RPE) present.

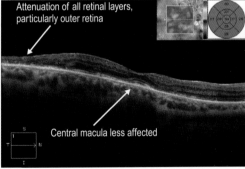

Attenuation of all retinal layers, particularly outer retina

Central macula less affected

Figure 15.1.2 OCT in advanced retinitis pigmentosa shows significant attenuation of all retinal layers, most notably of the outer retina, and worse temporally. OCT thickness map (inset) shows the degree of generalized retinal thinning throughout the macula. The central macula is affected to a lesser degree than the surrounding area.

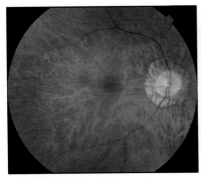

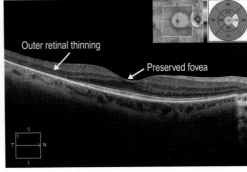

Figure 15.1.3 Color photograph of late-onset retinitis pigmentosa with mild disease shows mild pigment deposition and retinal thinning temporal to the macula. There is also unrelated peripapillary atrophy around the optic nerve.

Figure 15.1.4 OCT (corresponding to Figure 15.1.3) shows outer retinal thinning just outside the fovea. OCT thickness map (inset) shows a central island of normal retinal thickness with significant circumferential thinning outside of this area.

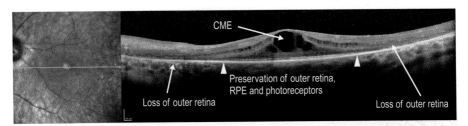

Figure 15.1.5 OCT of a patient with retinitis pigmentosa and associated cystoid macular edema. Despite the cystoid macular edema (CME), the outer retina and photoreceptors are relatively preserved in the central macula (between arrowheads) but are attenuated outside of this area.

15.2 | Stargardt Disease

Introduction: Stargardt disease is the most common inherited macular dystrophy. It is associated with mutations in the ABCA4 gene and is most commonly inherited in an autosomal recessive fashion. The disease has a wide spectrum of severity that accounts for a highly varied presentation.

Clinical Features: There are characteristic pisciform flecks or yellowish deposits that can be in the shape of a fish tail at the level of the retinal pigment epithelium (RPE). These deposits collect in the posterior pole, usually within the macula, but can be outside the arcades (Fig. 15.2.1). The peripapillary region is characteristically spared. Some cases show severe macular atrophy as the most prominent feature.

OCT Features: OCT confirms the **RPE as the location of the abnormal deposits** and reveals associated **outer retinal atrophy**, which may be present parafoveally (Fig. 15.2.2) or involve the fovea (Fig. 15.2.3). In more advanced stages of the disease, there is more widespread outer retinal atrophy that can lead to geographic atrophy (Fig. 15.2.4).

Ancillary Testing: Fluorescein angiography (FA) and fundus autofluorescence (FAF) can help in confirming the diagnosis. FA can show a characteristic dark choroid (Fig. 15.2.5), present in about 70% of cases. FAF highlights the abnormal RPE deposits and best demonstrates the peripapillary sparing (Figs. 15.2.6 and 15.2.7).

Treatment: No treatment is currently available.

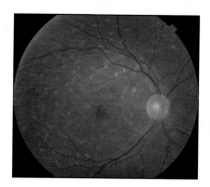

Figure 15.2.1 Color photograph shows numerous pisciform flecks throughout the posterior pole. There are also retinal pigment epithelium (RPE) abnormalities within the central macula.

Mild Stargardt disease

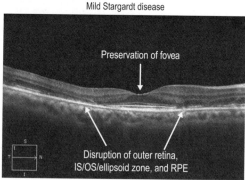

Preservation of fovea

Disruption of outer retina, IS/OS/ellipsoid zone, and RPE

Figure 15.2.2 OCT in a patient with mild Stargardt disease (corresponding to Figure 15.2.1) shows a characteristic bull's-eye maculopathy with preservation of the central fovea. There is disruption of the outer retina, IS–OS/ellipsoid zone, and retinal pigment epithelium (RPE) in a parafoveal ring.

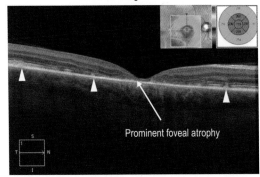

Moderate Stargardt disease

Prominent foveal atrophy

Figure 15.2.3 OCT in a patient with moderate Stargardt disease shows numerous hyper-reflective intra-RPE and sub-RPE deposits (arrowheads). There is diffuse loss of the outer retinal layers with prominent foveal atrophy, which is best demonstrated on the OCT thickness map (inset).

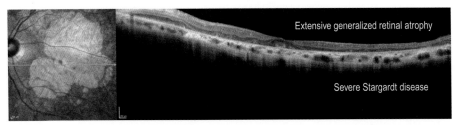

Extensive generalized retinal atrophy

Severe Stargardt disease

Figure 15.2.4 OCT in a patient with advanced Stargardt disease shows generalized outer retinal atrophy. There is corresponding negative shadowing of the underlying choroidal structures.

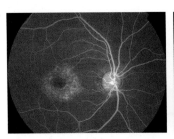
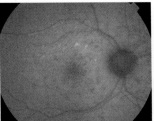
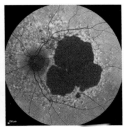

Figure 15.2.5 Mid-phase fluorescein angiography shows characteristic staining of central pisciform flecks in addition to a dark choroid.

Figure 15.2.6 Fundus autofluorescence (FAF) (corresponding to Figures 15.2.1 and 15.2.2) shows areas of both hyperautofluorescence and hypo-autofluorescence corresponding to pisciform flecks. The characteristic peripapillary sparing is well demonstrated.

Figure 15.2.7 Fundus autofluorescence (FAF) (corresponding to Figure 15.2.3) shows areas of both hyperautofluorescence and hypo-autofluorescence corresponding to pisciform flecks. There is a large area of profound central hypo-autofluorescence corresponding to geographic atrophy. Again, there is characteristic peripapillary sparing.

15.3 | Best Disease

Introduction: Best disease is due to a mutation in the BEST1 gene and is generally inherited in an autosomal dominant pattern with variable penetrance. BEST1 mutations are also associated with a variety of other phenotypes, including some cases of adult-onset foveomacular dystrophy, autosomal recessive bestrophinopathy, autosomal dominant vitreochoroidopathy, and some cases of rod–cone dystrophy.

Clinical Features: There are multiple clinical phenotypes, which represent different progressive stages of disease and include subclinical, vitelliform, pseudohypopyon, scrambled egg, and atrophic stages. The vitelliform stage has an egg yolk appearance of subretinal material, whereas the pseudohypopyon stage exhibits a gravitational layering of the yellow subretinal material with a fluid layer above (Fig. 15.3.1). The disease can be multifocal and asymmetric, leading to diagnostic uncertainty. Vision loss is most profound in the atrophic stage. Choroidal neovascularization (CNV) can rarely complicate the course in the atrophic stage.

OCT Features: OCT can distinguish differences between the various stages of Best disease. In the vitelliform stage, the **subretinal material** exhibits a mixture of both **hyper**-reflective and **hypo**reflective material. In the pseudohypopyon stage, there is a homogeneous, hypo-reflective layer above a hyper-reflective layer (Figs. 15.3.2 and 15.3.3) that can be confused with subretinal fluid secondary to CNV. This is best identified using a **vertical OCT scan**. The scrambled egg stage exhibits a mixture of retinal pigment epithelium (RPE) atrophy, pigment clumping, and subretinal fibrosis. The atrophic stage exhibits profound central atrophy of the outer retina and RPE.

Ancillary Testing: Fundus autofluorescence exhibits dramatic hyperautofluorescence (Fig. 15.3.4) and can be very helpful in assisting with the diagnosis. An electro-oculogram typically shows a reduced Arden ratio.

Treatment: No treatment is available except for the secondary CNV that can rarely occur.

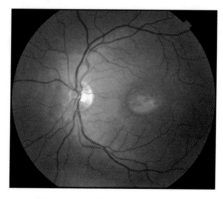

Figure 15.3.1 Color photograph of the pseudohypopyon stage of Best disease.

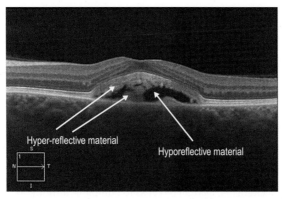

Figure 15.3.2 In the pseudohypopyon stage, a vertical OCT cut in the middle of the lesion would show a hyporeflective top layer (likely to be fluid) and a hyper-reflective bottom layer (likely to be more proteinaceous material) that are sharply demarcated. This example is a horizontal slice, which goes through both layers and shows a mix of both hypo- and hyper-reflective material in the subretinal space.

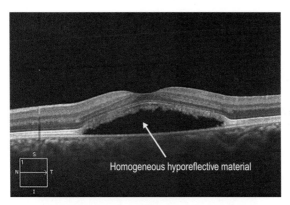

Figure 15.3.3 OCT may show homogeneous hyporeflective material in the subretinal space, which is most characteristic of the vitelliform or pseudohypopyon stages.

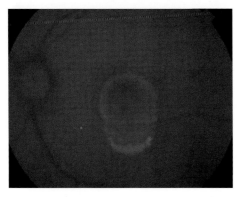

Figure 15.3.4 Fundus autofluorescence exhibits an extremely bright hyperautofluorescence pattern corresponding to lipofuscin deposits in the subretinal space.

15.4 Cone Dystrophy

Introduction: Cone dystrophy encompasses a heterogeneous group of inherited retinal dystrophies (IRDs) where isolated cone function is primarily affected.

Clinical Features: The clinical appearance can vary, but a central bull's-eye type maculopathy is most characteristic (Fig. 15.4.1). Early disease may present with a normal clinical examination. Symptoms include loss of visual acuity, color vision, and hemeralopia.

OCT Features: There is initially loss of the **outer retina and photoreceptors** within the **central macula** (Fig. 15.4.2). Over time, this can progress to **complete atrophy**. The peripheral macula and retinal periphery appear normal.

Ancillary Testing: Electrophysiologic testing shows a characteristic pattern where cone function is abnormal but the rod-isolated scotopic electroretinogram is normal or near normal. This is helpful to differentiate cone dystrophy from cone–rod retinitis pigmentosa.

Treatment: None.

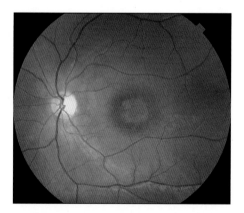

Figure 15.4.1 Color photograph of cone dystrophy shows a central bull's-eye maculopathy.

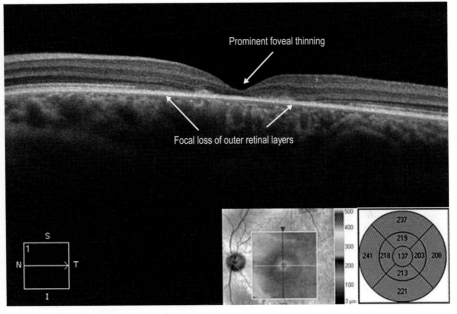

Figure 15.4.2 OCT (corresponding to Figure 15.4.1) shows focal central loss of the outer retinal layers (between arrowheads). There is prominent thinning in the fovea. The corresponding thickness map accentuates the degree of central macular thinning.

PART 6: Uveitis and Inflammatory Diseases

Section 16: Posterior Non-Infectious Uveitis 170

16.1 *Multifocal Choroditis* 170
Emily S. Levine

16.2 *Birdshot Chorioretinopathy* 174
Emily S. Levine

16.3 *Serpiginous Choroiditis* 178
Emily S. Levine

16.4 *Vogt–Koyanagi–Harada Disease* 182
Emily S. Levine

16.5 *Sympathetic Ophthalmia* 184
Emily S. Levine

16.6 *Posterior Scleritis* 186
Emily S. Levine

Section 17: Posterior Infection Uveitis 188

17.1 *Toxoplasma Chorioretinitis* 188
Eduardo Uchiyama

17.2 *Tuberculosis* 192
Eduardo Uchiyama

17.3 *Acute Syphilitic Posterior Placoid Chorioretinitis* 196
Eduardo Uchiyama

17.4 *Candida Albicans Endogenous Endophthalmitis* 198
Eduardo Uchiyama

17.5 *Acute Retinal Necrosis Syndrome* 200
Eduardo Uchiyama

16.1 | Multifocal Choroiditis

Introduction: Multifocal choroiditis with panuveitis (MCP) is a common, often idiopathic, usually bilateral, asymmetrical, chronic inflammatory disease occurring predominantly in myopic females in the second to sixth decades of life.

Clinical Features: Presentation of MCP is variable. Most patients complain of decreased visual acuity, but photopsia, floaters, blurring of central vision, scintillating scotoma, and enlargement of the blind spot can occur. Anterior segment inflammation may be present but is typically mild. Vitritis of variable severity and optic disc edema may be present. Multiple small, round to ovoid, pale lesions occur at the level of the outer retina, retinal pigment epithelium (RPE), and choroid, usually 50–350 µm in size, variable in number, and involve mainly the posterior pole (Fig. 16.1.1). Older lesions become pigmented and "punched-out" resembling histoplasmosis lesions. RPE metaplasia and choroidal neovascularization (peripapillary and macular) are common sequelae. Cystoid macular edema (CME), epiretinal membrane, and subretinal fibrosis may be seen later.

OCT Features: Active lesions show characteristic **transretinal hyper-reflectivity** and **drusen-like material** between the RPE and Bruch's membrane (Figs. 16.1.2 and 16.1.3). **Nodular collections beneath the RPE** appear to rupture with resulting **inflammatory infiltration** of the subretinal space and the outer retina. Slight **choroidal thickening, localized choroidal hyper-reflectivity** under the lesions, and **atrophy of the RPE and the retina** overlying the lesions and **vitreous cells** may be seen. Widespread loss of outer retinal architecture, **retinal thinning**, destructuring of the retinal layers, and **disappearance of IS–OS junction/ellipsoid layer** have also been seen in more advanced cases and may be associated with worse vision. Occasionally, choroidal neovascularization (CNV), **CME**, and **serous retinal detachments** may be seen. OCTA can help distinguish between an inflammatory lesion and a CNV (Fig. 16.1.4) by showing the presence or absence of choroidal neovascularization.

Ancillary Testing: On fluorescein angiography, active lesions show early hypofluorescence resulting from blockage and late staining (see Fig. 16.1.1). Atrophic lesions show early hyperfluorescence, which fades later, due to RPE window defects. Choroidal neovascularization or CME may be seen in the late phases.

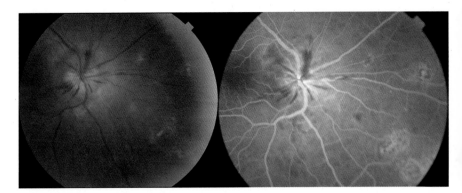

Figure 16.1.1 Color fundus photograph shows disc edema and hemorrhages and active lesions just nasal to the disc. The lesions are hypofluorescent in the intermediate stages of a fluorescein angiogram.

On fundus autofluorescence, macular hyperautofluorescence is seen in areas of active chorioretinitis delineating the diseased area.

On indocyanine green angiography, active lesions show hypofluorescence and may not be clinically visible. Old lesions show hypofluorescence throughout.

Visual field testing usually reveals an enlarged blind spot, but larger defects may be seen.

Treatment: Topical, periocular, and systemic corticosteroid treatment is the mainstay of therapy when the disease is active. Immunosuppressive therapy may be necessary in relentlessly progressive cases. Secondary choroidal neovascularization is not unusual and merits treatment with anti-vascular endothelial growth factor agents, laser photocoagulation, photodynamic therapy, corticosteroids, or a combination thereof.

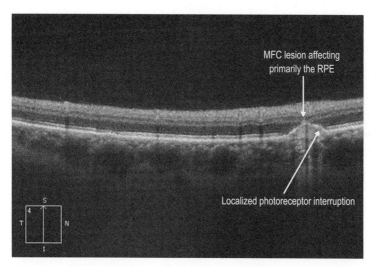

Figure 16.1.2 OCT through an active choroidal lesion demonstrates solid retinal pigment epithelium (RPE) detachments or drusen-like deposits below the RPE with some overlying RPE and outer retinal atrophy. Lesions with transretinal hyper-reflectivity are also seen.

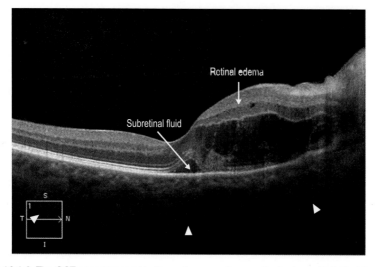

Figure 16.1.3 The OCT scan temporal to the optic nerve shows retinal edema. Note that the choroid appears thickened and the posterior choroido–scleral border is not visible (arrowheads).

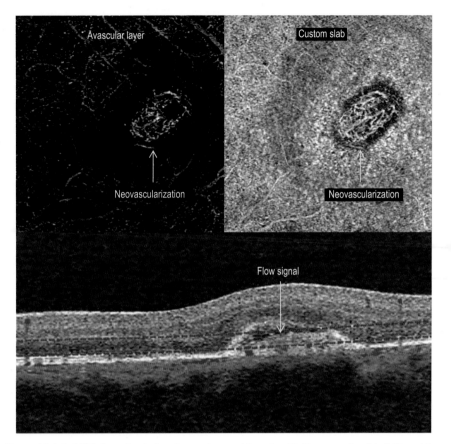

Figure 16.1.4 OCTA through a lesion shows abnormal flow signal in the avascular slab (left), and the B-scan reveals flow pixels in the lesion in this slab (lower). A custom segmentation shows a detailed view of the neovascular network.

16.2 | Birdshot Chorioretinopathy

Introduction: Birdshot retinochoroidopathy, also called vitiliginous chorioretinitis, is a rare bilateral posterior uveitis affecting usually healthy adults between the third and sixth decades of life with a female preponderance. An autoimmune pathogenesis has been suggested with reactivity to the retinal S antigen. There is a strong association with HLA-A29 (>90% of cases). HLA-B44 is also positive in many cases.

Clinical Features: Decreased vision, photopsias, floaters, nyctalopia, and decreased color vision are frequent symptoms. There is minimal to no anterior uveitis with mild vitritis. Multifocal depigmented cream-colored retinal pigment epithelium lesions less than one disc diameter in size are scattered throughout the fundus, although these may be absent or very subtle in the early stages of the disease (Fig. 16.2.1). Retinal phlebitis, narrowing and sheathing of retinal vasculature, disc edema, optic atrophy, cystoid macular edema, choroidal neovascularization, and epiretinal membrane may also develop. It is invariably bilateral.

OCT Features: Line scan of the macula may show the typical features of birdshot: **epiretinal membrane formation** and **macular edema** (Fig. 16.2.2). **Subretinal fluid** may be seen in severe cases of macular edema. In chronic cases, the macula is **diffusely thin** and **disruption of the IS–OS segment/ellipsoid layer** with **disorganization of the inner retinal layers** and **retinal pigment epithelium atrophy** may be seen (Fig. 16.2.3). Focal and generalized **loss of the IS–OS junction/ellipsoid layer**, loss of retinal architecture, and **outer retinal hyper-reflective foci** overlying the lesions are typical. **Generalized thinning** of the choroid and outer retina in long-standing cases and **hyporeflective suprachoroidal space** are other features. Extramacular and enhanced depth or swept-source OCT images provide greater information than regular macular scans, because the choroidal lesions themselves can be scanned. OCTA is not routinely used for the diagnosis of birdshot but may show telangiectasia, capillary dilatations and loops, and increased intercapillary space in the retinal vasculature (Fig. 16.2.4). OCTA also reveals multifocal dark spots of hypoperfusion in the choriocapillaris and deeper in the choroid that sometimes correlate spatially with hypopigmented fundus lesions (Fig. 16.2.5).

Ancillary Testing: Diagnosis is based on clinical features. On fluorescein angiography (FA), birdshot lesions may block dye in the early phases and stain in the late phases. All lesions seen on clinical examination may not be evident on FA. There may be retinal vascular leakage, perifoveal capillary leakage, disc edema, staining, and late cystoid macular edema. Occasionally, choroidal neovascularization may be seen at the site of old lesions. Indocyanine green angiography reveals early hypofluorescent spots and possible diffuse late leakage. Many more spots may be seen on indocyanine green angiography than on FA, further consolidating the theory that this is primarily a choroidal disease.

Electroretinogram shows depressed rod and cone function with a decreased b-wave amplitude and increased latency of the b-wave compared with the a-wave, which is relatively preserved. The b-wave may eventually be extinguished in severe cases. The 30 Hz flicker response is delayed with increased implicit times.

HLA testing (HLA-A29) is positive in 80–100% of patients.

Treatment: The mainstay of treatment is periocular and systemic steroids. Steroid-sparing treatments used include cyclosporine, azathioprine, methotrexate, infliximab, immunoglobulins, and mycophenolate mofetil. Targeted treatments are being studied.

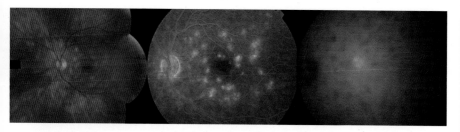

Figure 16.2.1 Characteristic fundus photograph of a patient with birdshot with hypopigmented lesions noted extending into the mid-periphery. Late frames of the fluorescein angiography show hyperfluorescence and late-frame indocyanine green angiography shows the lesions as hypocyanescent spots with some diffuse hypercyanescence.

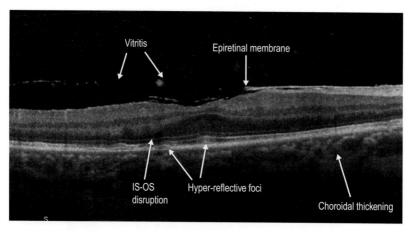

Figure 16.2.2 OCT scan shows vitritis, epiretinal membrane formation, and disruption of the IS–OS/ellipsoid layer with some inner retinal disorganization.

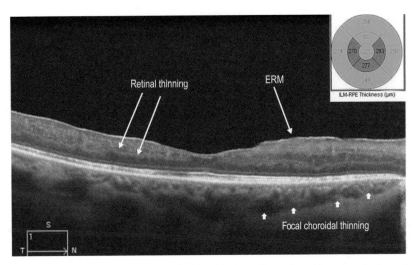

Figure 16.2.3 OCT in late-stage birdshot showing thinning of the retina with preferential loss of outer retinal layers.

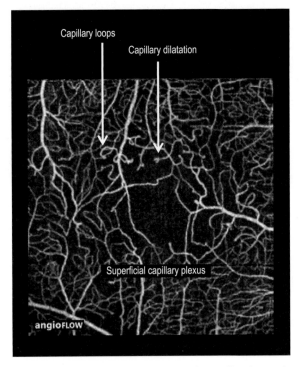

Figure 16.2.4 OCTA of the superficial capillary plexus showing capillary loops, abnormally tortuous vessels, and capillary dilatations. (Courtesy Talisa de Carlo, MD.)

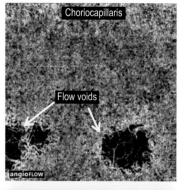

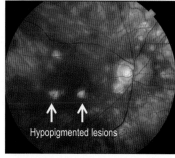

Figure 16.2.5 OCTA of the choriocapillaris revealing decreased flow signal at two lesions indicated by arrows in the respective color fundus photograph. (Courtesy Talisa de Carlo, MD.)

16.3 | Serpiginous Choroiditis

Introduction: Serpiginous choroiditis, also known as helicoid or geographic choroidopathy, is a rare, idiopathic inflammatory disease affecting the retinal pigment epithelium, outer retina, and the inner choroid. It is slightly more common in men between 30 and 70 years of age with no predilection for race. It usually occurs in otherwise healthy individuals.

Clinical Features: The most common complaints are blurring of vision and central or paracentral scotomata, but occasionally it is diagnosed asymptomatically on routine examination. Anterior segment inflammation is usually mild, and the vitreous may be clear or show minimal inflammation. The disease can be classified on the basis of clinical presentation as:

▸ Peripapillary
▸ Macular
▸ Ampiginous

Lesions most commonly start in the peripapillary region (Fig. 16.3.1). Active lesions are yellow to grayish with associated overlying retinal edema. These spread in a centripetal, helicoid, map-like or snake-like pattern from the initial area of involvement. Active lesions become atrophic in weeks to months, with atrophy of the retinal pigment epithelium, choriocapillaris, and choroid. New lesions arise at the edge of the atrophic ones. Choroidal neovascularization, subretinal hemorrhage, and serous retinal detachment can complicate the course. The disease is typically chronic and remitting with quiescent periods of up to several years between active episodes.

OCT Features: The characteristic active lesion of serpiginous choroiditis shows **hyper-reflectivity and thickening of the outer retina**, and **increased reflectance of the choroid**. This has been referred to as the **'waterfall' effect** (Figs. 16.3.2 and 16.3.3). There is also **disruption of the photoreceptor inner and outer segment junction** in both active and inactive lesions (Figs. 16.3.2 and 16.3.3). There is complete absence of flow signal in the choriocapillaris of active lesions on OCTA. Swept source OCTA reveals atrophic areas of the choriocapillaris with greater visibility of large choroidal vessels in inactive lesions.

Ancillary Testing: Visual field examination reveals central or paracentral scotoma. Fluorescein angiography of the active lesions show early hypofluorescence and late hyper-fluorescence in a typical geographic pattern. Retinal vessels may stain adjacent to the active lesions. Old lesions show window defects and late staining (see Fig. 16.3.1D–F). Indocyanine green angiography reveals choroidal non-perfusion (see Fig. 16.3.1C).

Fundus hyperautofluorescence provides a clear demarcation of the retinal pigment epithelium damage in acute lesions. Scarring of the lesions causes decreased autofluorescence.

Treatment: Periocular and systemic corticosteroids have been used to treat acute episodes (Fig. 16.3.4), and long-term steroid-sparing therapy such as cyclosporine, azathioprine, cyclophosphamide, interferon alpha-2a, or infliximab is needed to prevent recurrence.

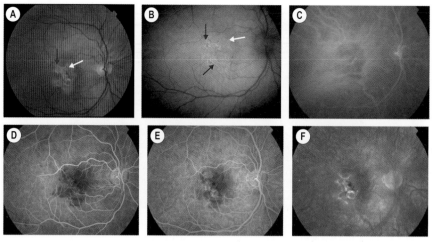

Figure 16.3.1 Color photograph (A) and autofluorescence (B) show macular serpiginous, with old inactive lesion (red arrows) and active lesion at the margin (white arrow). Indocyanine green angiography (C) shows choroidal hypofluorescence consistent with areas of activity. Fluorescein angiography (D–F) shows early hypofluorescence and late hyper-fluorescence.

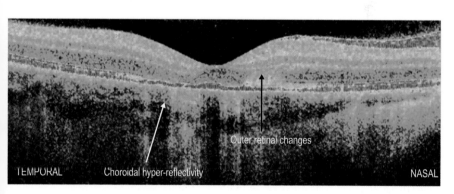

Figure 16.3.2 OCT shows choroidal hyper-reflectivity (white arrow), outer retinal thickening (black arrow), and disruption of the ellipsoid IS–OS layer.

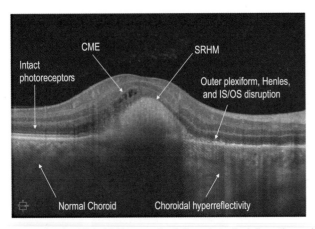

Figure 16.3.3 B-scan showing choroidal hyper-reflectivity, outer retinal disruption, subretinal hyper-reflective material (SRHM), and cystoid macular edema (CME).

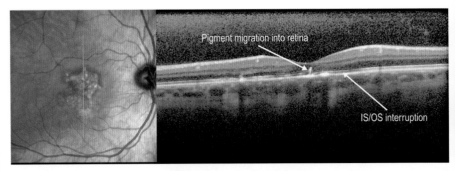

Figure 16.3.4 The same patient from Figure 16.3.2 after treatment with steroids. Note resolution of the choroidal hyper-reflectivity and retinal thickening.

16.4 | Vogt–Koyanagi–Harada Disease

Introduction: Vogt–Koyanagi–Harada (VKH) disease is a rare, bilateral, chronic, idiopathic, granulomatous panuveitis. It occurs predominantly in women, usually between 30 and 50 years old, with a propensity for dark-pigmented races: Asians, Hispanics, Native Americans, and Asian Indians. An immune reaction to uveal melanocytes has been proposed as the mechanism, but the cause largely remains unknown.

Clinical Features: Initially, VKH was classified as two separate diseases:

▸ Vogt–Koyanagi syndrome: comprising chronic anterior uveitis, alopecia, poliosis, vitiligo, and dysacousia.
▸ Harada's disease: comprising bilateral posterior, exudative uveitis, and neurological features.
Considering the considerable overlap in the features, the term *VKH* disease is now used.

At onset, patients may experience flu-like symptoms, central nervous system signs, optic neuropathy, sensitivity of hair and skin to touch, perilimbal vitiligo, alopecia, vitiligo poliosis, and auditory signs. Blurred vision, photophobia, conjunctival hyperemia, and ocular pain also occur. Bilateral anterior and exudative posterior uveitis is typical. Shallow, serous retinal detachments are seen at the posterior pole with underlying choroidal infiltrates (Fig. 16.4.1). The optic disc is edematous and hyperemic.

With resolution of the uveitis and retinal detachments, a gradual depigmented appearance of the choroid (sunset-glow fundus) may develop.

OCT Features: OCT reveals **serous retinal detachments** at the macula. The **subretinal fluid** may reveal a higher optical density than the vitreous, suggesting a higher level of protein content (Figs. 16.4.2 and 16.4.3). Inner retinal layers are typically well preserved with **cystic changes** and complex infolding in the outer retinal layers. **Subretinal fibrinoid deposits** are seen, which may later evolve into **subretinal fibrosis**. **Vitreoretinal interface alterations** with cellular deposits may also be seen. There may be alteration and **thickening of the IS–OS junction/ellipsoid layer, RPE and choroidal folds**, and **thickening of the choroid**, sometimes to an extreme degree. Enhanced depth imaging and swept source OCT will show significant choroidal thickening, which resolves when treated. OCTA is not routinely used in the testing of VKH, but preliminary studies show multiple dark foci of hypoperfusion in the choriocapillaris during the acute phase that decrease in number and size with treatment.

Ancillary Testing: On fluorescein angiography, active disease with subretinal exudation appears as multiple hyperfluorescent dots at the retinal pigment epithelium (RPE) level, which gradually enlarge and coalesce as the dye accumulates in the subretinal space. With resolution of the exudative phase, these features are no longer visualized. The chronic phase is characterized by diffuse scattered hyper-fluorescent dots corresponding to window defects at the RPE level.

On fundus autofluorescence, serous detachments are observed to be hypoautofluorescent, due to blockage. Hypoautofluorescent multiple, granular dots are seen after resolution, which correspond to the window defects on FA.

On indocyanine green angiography, active disease is characterized by choroidal stromal vasculature hyper-fluorescence and leakage, disc hyper-fluorescence, hypofluorescent dots, and indistinct, fuzzy large choroidal vessels with decreased dye filling.

▸ Ultrasonography: ultrasound is helpful if the posterior segment is not visible, and reveals diffusely thickened posterior choroid with low to medium reflectivity, serous retinal detachments, vitritis, and thickened sclera or episclera.
▸ Cerebrospinal fluid analysis: cerebrospinal fluid pleocytosis and elevated protein levels are seen.
Treatment: Topical, periocular, and systemic steroids are instituted as therapy, along with topical cycloplegics. In chronic or non-responsive cases or when side effects from steroids are severe, other agents are used including cyclosporine, chlorambucil, cyclophosphamide, azathioprine, or infliximab.

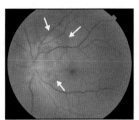
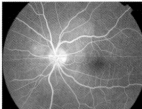
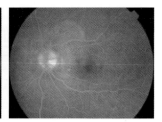

Figure 16.4.1 Color fundus photograph of a patient with Vogt–Koyanagi–Harada shows the classic exudative posterior pole detachment (arrows). Intermediate-stage fluorescein angiography shows multiple hyper-fluorescent spots at the choroidal level and some diffuse pooling of dye in the subretinal space. Late-stage fluorescein angiography shows disc hyperemia and staining with pooling of dye in the serous retinal detachment.

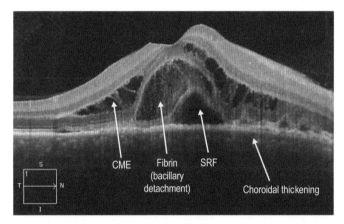

Figure 16.4.2 OCT scan through the macular detachment in a patient with Vogt–Koyanagi–Harada shows the turbid subretinal fluid (SRF) with fibrin deposition. There are outer retinal cystic changes seen. The retina is thickened. *CME*, Cystoid macular edema.

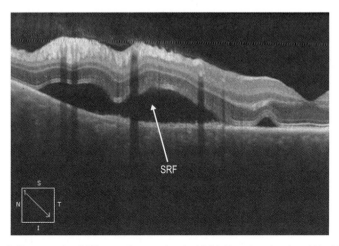

Figure 16.4.3 Extramacular OCT scan shows subretinal fluid. Note that the choroid is thickened and the choroidoscleral border is not visible. *SRF*, Subretinal fluid.

16.5 | Sympathetic Ophthalmia

Introduction: Sympathetic ophthalmia is an exceedingly rare, bilateral diffuse granulomatous uveitis that develops after ocular penetrating trauma or surgery. Inflammation in the contralateral, unaffected eye develops days to years after the event, but usually occurs within 3 months of the injury.

Epidemiology: Sympathetic ophthalmia is rare, affecting 0.2–0.5% of all traumatic penetrating eye injuries and 0.007% of patients after ocular surgery featuring a penetrating incision. The risk after pars plana vitrectomy is 0.01%.

Clinical Features: Clinically, patients present with a bilateral severe, unremitting granulomatous panuveitis. There may be associated hypotony, small depigmented nodules at the level of the retinal pigment epithelium (Dalen-Fuch's nodules), choroidal thickening, and serous retinal detachments (Fig. 16.5.1). Signs of prior injury or surgery in one eye are present.

OCT Features: OCT findings include **posterior choroidal thickening** and accumulation of **turbid subretinal fluid** with deposition of fibrin and/or fibrinous bands in the subretinal fluid (Fig. 16.5.2). **Macular edema** may also be seen. In later stages of sympathetic ophthalmia, there is retinal and retinal pigment epithelium **atrophy and thinning** with **transmission defects** noted (Fig. 16.5.3).

Treatment: Sympathetic ophthalmia can be prevented by enucleation of a blind, injured eye within 2 weeks after the trauma. Even after the onset of sympathetic ophthalmia, it may be of help to enucleate the eye that was previously injured. Once sympathetic ophthalmia is established in the contralateral eye, the mainstay of treatment consists of systemic anti-inflammatory agents such as oral corticosteroids or other immunosuppressive agents. More recently, treatments with local injections of corticosteroids in combination with or without systemic therapy and intravitreal injections of infliximab have been reported.

Severe cases of sympathetic ophthalmia may be refractory to treatment.

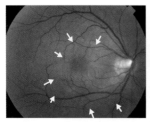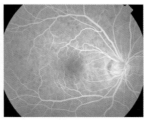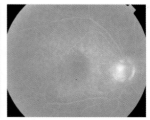

Figure 16.5.1 Red-free photo of a macular serous detachment associated with sympathetic ophthalmia. The fluorescein angiogram shows pooling in the subretinal space associated with a serous retinal detachment. The left-most image is a red-free photo of a macular serous detachment (outlined by white arrows) associated with sympathetic ophthalmia. The middle and right images are fluorescein angiograms showing pooling in the subretinal space associated with a serous retinal detachment.

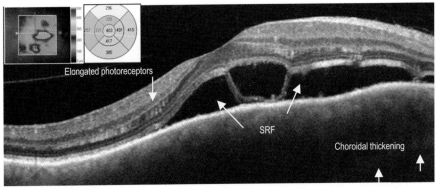

Figure 16.5.2 OCT scan through the macula shows a serous retinal detachment with fibrin deposits and bands (arrows). The choroid is thickened (short arrows) and the photoreceptors appear elongated. The thickness map shows thickening in the region with the serous retinal detachment. *SRF*, subretinal fluid.

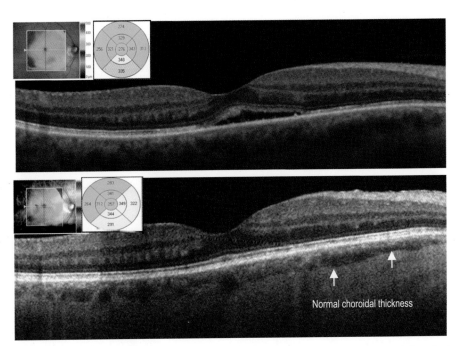

Figure 16.5.3 Sequential post-treatment OCTs show resolution of the subretinal fluid and the retinal detachment. Note that the choroidal thickness is reduced (arrows).

16.6 | Posterior Scleritis

Introduction: Posterior scleritis is uncommon inflammation of the sclera occurring posterior to the insertion of the rectus muscles. Posterior scleritis can occur in isolation or in association with anterior scleritis. There is strong female preponderance resulting from its association with autoimmune disorders. Scleritis has been associated with many systemic diseases, but the strongest association is with rheumatoid arthritis. It usually occurs in the fourth to sixth decades of life. Infectious scleritis has also been reported, but infectious posterior scleritis is rare.

Clinical Features: Common presenting features are pain, tenderness, blurred vision, proptosis, and pain or restriction of eye movements. One-third of patients will have no pain. Common findings include retinal striae, exudative retinal detachment, and choroidal thickening and detachments (Fig. 16.6.1). Less common manifestations are macular and disc edema, subretinal mass, hemorrhages, and exudation. Diagnosis may be difficult in the absence of anterior scleritis.

OCT Features: Cystoid macular edema can occur, but **serous macular and retinal detachments** are most common. The choroid may be **thickened** on enhanced depth imaging scanning (Figs. 16.6.2 and 16.6.3).

Ancillary Testing: Fluorescein angiography is strikingly similar to that seen in Vogt–Koyanagi–Harada disease, with subretinal leakage points that coalesce in the late phases. B-scan ultrasonography reveals fluid in the sub-Tenon's space that may manifest as the classic T-sign. Scleral thickening is also seen. Exudative retinal detachments may also be visualized. Computed tomography or magnetic resonance imaging scan of the orbits may show diffuse thickening of the sclera (the ring 360 degree sign on computed tomography scanning).

Treatment: Systemic associations should be ruled out. Non-steroidal anti-inflammatory drug therapy, oral corticosteroid therapy, or, in recalcitrant or recurrent cases, immunosuppressive drugs are effective treatments.

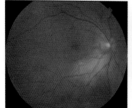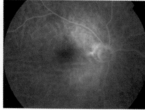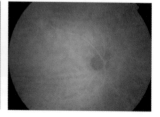

Figure 16.6.1 Fundus photograph of a patient with posterior scleritis showing some obscuration of choroidal detail and subtle choroidal folds better seen on the accompanying fluorescein angiography and indocyanine green angiography.

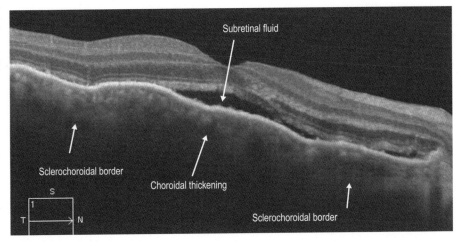

Figure 16.6.2 OCT scanning through the macula reveals a serous macular detachment. There is choroidal thickening seen and the posterior extent of the choroid cannot be visualized on the OCT scan.

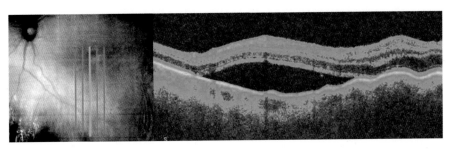

Figure 16.6.3 OCT scan showing relatively flat macula but with gravitation of the exudative retinal detachment inferiorly.

17.1 | Toxoplasma Chorioretinitis

Introduction: Toxoplasmosis is a zoonotic infection caused by the protozoan parasite *Toxoplasma gondii*. It is the most common cause of posterior uveitis and focal retinitis. The disease typically affects immunocompetent individuals.

Clinical Features: In recurrent cases, there is a characteristic focus of active chorioretinitis with overlying vitritis adjacent to a pigmented chorioretinal scar (Fig. 17.1.1). Associated retinal vasculitis may be present. The disease is almost always unilateral. Primary infection may present with a similar appearance in the absence of a pigmented scar (Fig. 17.1.2). Multifocality and bilaterality are rare, except in immunocompromised individuals. In elderly patients, a severe form of toxoplasmosis that is relentlessly progressive, resembling acute retinal necrosis, can occur.

OCT Features: Peripheral lesions are often not amenable to imaging with OCT, but if located within or near the macula, OCT reveals **thickening and distortion of all the retinal layers** and the RPE (Fig. 17.1.3) within the area of active chorioretinitis. **Vitreous opacities** are sometimes seen over areas of active retinitis, which indicate disease activity. Kyrieleis **plaques** are a non-specific finding that can be present **overlying retinal blood vessels** in the setting of vasculitis from toxoplasmic chorioretinitis. These appear as hyper-reflective, round outpouchings or plaque-like deposits on the surface of both arteries and veins (Fig. 17.1.4). Following the acute stage of active chorioretinitis, full-thickness retinal necrosis occurs with **cavitary loss of retinal tissue**, eventually leaving varying degrees of subretinal scarring (Fig. 17.1.5) Choroidal neovascularization can occur secondarily from toxoplasmosis scars, and OCT can show associated intraretinal and subretinal fluid.

Ancillary Testing: Fluorescein angiography can be helpful but is not necessary. Clinical examination is typically enough to confirm the diagnosis. If the diagnosis is in doubt, intraocular fluid sampling with polymerase chain reaction testing can be confirmative.

Treatment: The disease course is most frequently self-limited, and proof of treatment efficacy is lacking. Disease threatening the macula or optic nerve is more apt to be treated. Numerous strategies of various oral and intravitreal antimicrobial agents have been used.

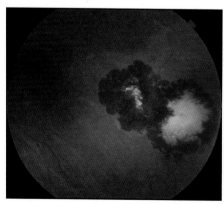

Figure 17.1.1 Color photograph of a typical toxoplasmosis chorioretinal scar with resolving active retinitis.

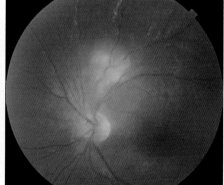

Figure 17.1.2 Color photograph of primary toxoplasmosis chorioretinitis superior to the optic nerve in a 14-year-old female who had congenital toxoplasmosis infection.

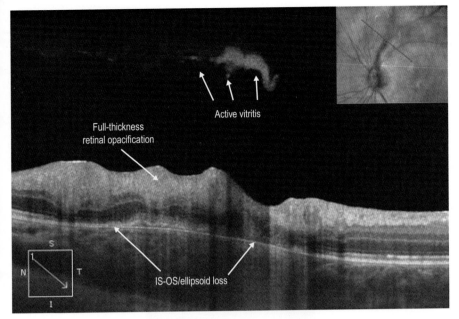

Figure 17.1.3 OCT using enhanced depth imaging protocol (corresponding to Figure 17.1.2) shows distortion and thickening of all retinal layers in the area of active chorioretinitis. The inner retinal layers are more involved and are hyper-reflective. There are patchy areas of IS–OS/ellipsoid zone and retinal pigment epithelium loss. Vitreous opacities are visible overlying the retinal lesion, indicative of active disease.

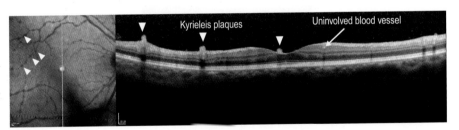

Figure 17.1.4 OCT vertical line scan and corresponding infrared image through Kyrieleis plaques reveals hyper-reflective circular opacities (arrowheads) overlying both retinal arterioles and venules.

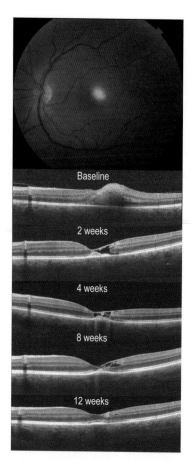

Figure 17.1.5 Color photograph of acute toxoplasmosis in the macula (top) with corresponding OCT and subsequent OCTs over a 3-month period. The acute lesion shows full-thickness retinal involvement with thickening and disorganization. By 2 weeks, there is a sizable empty cavity within the retina as a result of necrosis and lost tissue. This necrotic region somewhat reorganizes by 12 weeks overlying an area of subretinal fibrosis.

17.2 | Tuberculosis

Introduction: *Mycobacterium tuberculosis* can infect many extrapulmonary organs, including the eyes. It is a common infectious cause of uveitis in certain, mostly tropical, countries. HIV-infected patients are particularly at risk of disease.

Clinical Features: Ocular manifestations include choroidal granuloma, choroiditis, chorioretinitis, optic nerve infiltration, and uveitis (Figs. 17.2.1 and 17.2.2). Choroidal involvement can cause changes in the posterior pole, similar to that seen in serpiginous choroiditis, or can be multifocal in nature. Multiple old, inactive associated chorioretinal scars are suggestive of tuberculosis.

OCT Features: OCT is particularly useful to image tuberculosis involvement of the retina and choroid. Infiltration in the subretinal space and choroid by a homogeneous material of medium to high reflectivity is typical early in the disease course (Fig. 17.2.3). There can also be associated subretinal fluid. Resolving chorioretinitis can leave varying degrees of retinal and choroidal destruction along with deposition of hyper-reflective subretinal material (Figs. 17.2.4 and 17.2.5).

Ancillary Testing: Tuberculin skin testing, interferon-gamma release assays, and chest radiography can be used to help in the diagnosis. Fluorescein angiography and fundus autofluorescence can aid in identifying multifocal serpiginous-like choroiditis typical in tubercular ocular disease (Fig. 17.2.6). Referral for a complete medical evaluation is warranted if tuberculosis is suspected.

Treatment: No directed ocular therapy is indicated. There are numerous systemic anti-tubercular therapeutic agents available. Treatment should be coordinated by an infectious disease specialist.

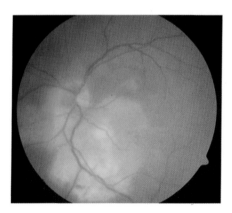

Figure 17.2.1 Color photograph of active tubercular chorioretinitis involving the macula and optic nerve. (Courtesy Alay S. Banker, MD.)

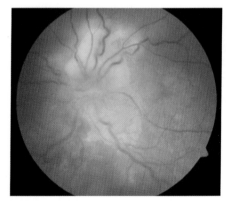

Figure 17.2.2 Color photograph of active tubercular chorioretinitis (superior to optic nerve) and resolving chorioretinitis (in macula). (Courtesy Alay S. Banker, MD.)

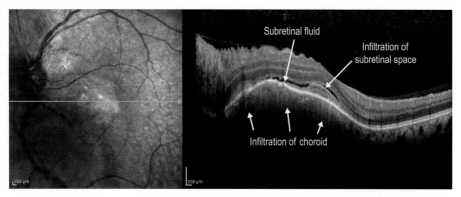

Figure 17.2.3 OCT (corresponding to Figure 17.2.1) shows homogeneous infiltration of the choroid causing an irregular, dome-shaped elevation of the overlying retinal pigment epithelium (RPE) and retina. There is also infiltration of the subretinal space with a homogeneous material of medium reflectivity and associated subretinal fluid. (Courtesy Alay S. Banker, MD.)

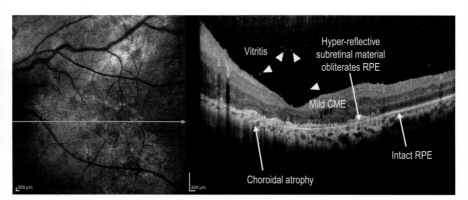

Figure 17.2.4 OCT (corresponding to Figure 17.2.2) of resolving tubercular chorioretinitis shows atrophy of the choroid. The subretinal space has a thin layer of hyper-reflective material that has obliterated the retinal pigment epithelium (RPE), as there is negative shadowing ending abruptly where the RPE is intact. Other features include mild cystoid macular edema (CME) and small hyper-reflective deposits in the vitreous (arrowheads), which probably represent vitreous infiltration by tuberculosis organisms or secondary inflammation. (Courtesy Alay S. Banker, MD.)

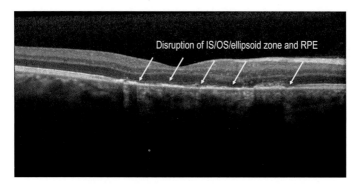

Figure 17.2.5 OCT of serpiginous-like choroiditis due to tuberculosis shows extensive disruption of the IS/OS/ellipsoid zone and retinal pigment epithelium (RPE). (Courtesy Eduardo Uchiyama, MD.)

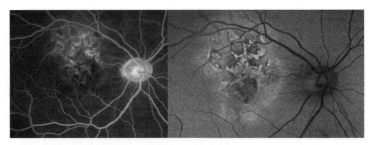

Figure 17.2.6 Fluorescein angiography (left) and fundus autofluorescence (right) (corresponding to Figure 17.2.5) show patterns typical of multifocal serpiginous-like choroiditis due to tuberculosis. (Courtesy Eduardo Uchiyama, MD.)

17.3 Acute Syphilitic Posterior Placoid Chorioretinitis

Introduction: Ocular syphilis is a rare manifestation of disease caused by the spirochete *Treponema pallidum*. Intraocular involvement can occur at any stage of infection. There is high correlation with co-infection of human immunodeficiency virus type 1.

Clinical Features: Ocular involvement typically manifests as posterior uveitis with chorioretinitis. Acute syphilitic posterior placoid chorioretinitis (ASPPC) is a specific and characteristic manifestation of ocular syphilis. A singular yellow-colored, circular, deep retinal plaque located in the macula is characteristically present (Fig. 17.3.1). The lesions may be multifocal and subtle. Bilaterality occurs in about half of affected patients.

OCT Features: Much like the disease itself, the OCT findings can vary. Focal and patchy loss of the **IS–OS/ellipsoid zone** with intermixed hyper-reflective nodular lesions of the retinal pigment epithelium (RPE) are the most common and typical features of ASPPC (Fig. 17.3.2). The **external limiting membrane** is typically disrupted focally over the nodular RPE lesions. Punctate hyper-reflectivity within the choroid may also be present. Serous retinal detachments involving the macula are uncommon, transient, and occur in about 10% of cases in the acute phase (Fig. 17.3.3). Following appropriate treatment, acute OCT findings normalize promptly (Figs. 17.3.2 and 17.3.3).

Ancillary Testing: Fluorescein angiography usually shows a central hypofluorescent area corresponding to the plaque early, occasionally with leopard spotting, followed by progressive hyperfluorescence later (Fig. 17.3.4). Late staining from the retinal vessels and optic nerve, even outside areas of retinal whitening, is typical. Indocyanine green angiography typically shows hypofluorescence in both early and late stages.

Treatment: Prompt treatment with intravenous penicillin G (2.4 million units daily for 14 days) is indicated. Testing should be performed for both human immunodeficiency virus and neurosyphilis.

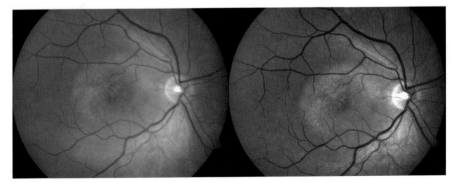

Figure 17.3.1 Color (left) and red-free (right) photographs of typical acute syphilitic posterior placoid chorioretinitis (ASPPC) shows a yellowish, circular deep retinal plaque involving the macula. (Courtesy Lana Rifkin, MD.)

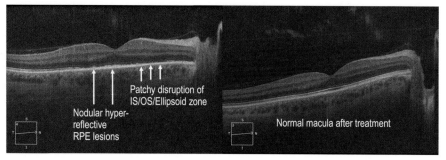

Patchy disruption of
IS/OS/Ellipsoid zone

Nodular hyper-
reflective
RPE lesions

Normal macula after treatment

Figure 17.3.2 OCT (corresponding to Fig. 17.3.1) of acute ASPPC (left) shows characteristic patchy loss of the IS/OS/ellipsoid zone and hyper-reflective nodular RPE lesions. One month following intravenous ceftriaxone therapy (right), the macular appearance normalized. (From Goldman, D. R. (2018). Acute syphilitic posterior placoid chorioretinitis. In: D.R. Goldman, N.K. Waheed, & J.S. Duker (Eds.), *Atlas of retinal OCT: Optical coherence tomography* (pp. 121–123). Philadelphia: Elsevier. Courtesy Lana Rifkin, MD.)

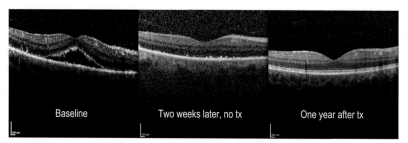

Baseline

Two weeks later, no tx

One year after tx

Figure 17.3.3 OCT of acute syphilitic posterior placoid chorioretinitis (ASPPC) (left) shows subretinal fluid beneath the fovea, a finding seen in the minority of cases. Two weeks later but prior to initiation of treatment (middle), the macular appearance is more typical of ASPPC with nodular hyper-reflective RPE lesions. One year following intravenous penicillin therapy (right), the macular appearance normalized. (Courtesy Eduardo Uchiyama, MD.)

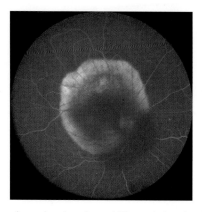

Figure 17.3.4 Fluorescein angiography of acute syphilitic posterior placoid chorioretinitis (ASPPC) shows diffuse hyper-fluorescence delineating sharp borders of the plaque-like lesion. (Courtesy Eduardo Uchiyama, MD.)

17.4 | *Candida Albicans* Endogenous Endophthalmitis

Introduction: *Candida albicans* is the most common pathogen responsible for fungal endophthalmitis. Intravenous drug use, in-dwelling catheters, and immunocompromised host status are risk factors for infection.

Clinical Features: The clinical appearance of *C. albicans* endogenous endophthalmitis is very characteristic. The lesions typically consist of small areas of chorioretinitis involving the posterior pole, are creamy-white in color and have fairly well-defined borders (Fig. 17.4.1). Overlying vitritis is typical, often in a "string of pearls" arrangement (Fig. 17.4.2). Affected patients may not necessarily be systemically ill.

OCT Features: OCT can identify characteristic features of fungal chorioretinitis. *C. albicans* retinal infiltrates are **located superficially** in the retina. They are **hyper-reflective, dome-shaped elevations** overlying the inner retina (Fig. 17.4.3). They obscure the underlying retina due to shadowing. **Poor signal strength** is common because of the presence of overlying inflammatory debris in the vitreous cavity. Active lesions resolve following appropriate antifungal treatment, leaving varying degrees of focal retinal disorganization and choroidal atrophy.

Ancillary Testing: Diagnosis is typically made by clinical exam alone. Vitreous biopsy can help confirm the diagnosis.

Treatment: Various antifungal agents are available and can be administered via oral, intravenous, and intravitreal routes dependent on disease severity.

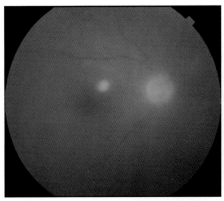

Figure 17.4.1 Color photograph shows a creamy-white, fluffy, well-circumscribed retinal infiltrate in the superonasal macula. There is moderate overlying vitritis.

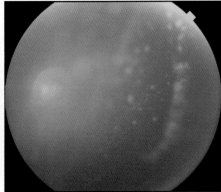

Figure 17.4.2 Color photograph shows many small yellow vitreous opacities connected by inflammatory debris in a characteristic "string of pearls" arrangement.

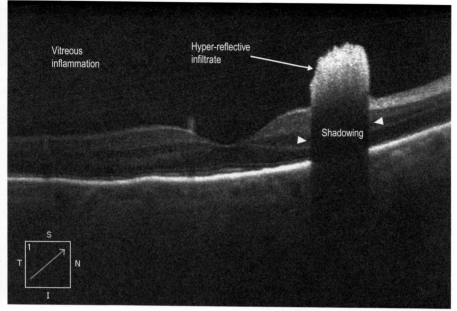

Figure 17.4.3 OCT shows a well-circumscribed, hyper-reflective, dome-shaped elevation overlying the retina (arrow). There is dense shadowing (between arrowheads) obscuring the underlying structures. The overall signal quality of the scan is poor because of moderate vitreous inflammation.

17.5 | Acute Retinal Necrosis Syndrome

Introduction: Acute retinal necrosis (ARN) syndrome, also known as acute herpetic retinitis, is a rare disorder occurring most commonly in immunocompetent adults. The most common etiologic agent is varicella zoster virus, followed by herpes simplex viruses (types 1 and 2) and, very rarely, cytomegalovirus.

Clinical Features: ARN commonly presents with multifocal peripheral areas of full-thickness retinal necrosis in well-circumscribed patches that rapidly coalesce in a circumferential pattern (Fig. 17.5.1). There is an associated brisk intraocular inflammatory reaction and an occlusive vasculitis that primarily affect the retinal arteries. Vitritis is universal, and a mild anterior chamber reaction with keratic precipitates is typical. Elevated intraocular pressure is not unusual. Without treatment, spread is rapid and may also involve the fellow eye.

OCT Features: In cases where the macula is not directly involved clinically but is threatened, OCT shows subclinical disease involvement (Fig. 17.5.2), which can be useful for prognostic purposes. Disease activity beyond the clinically evident area of involvement (or leading edge) is typical of this condition. In acute, active retinitis there is hyper-reflectivity and disorganization of all retinal layers (Fig. 17.5.3). Associated subretinal fluid, choroidal thickening, and overlying vitreous inflammation may be present. After regression of retinitis, there is significant atrophy/attenuation of all retinal layers (Fig. 17.5.4).

Ancillary Testing: Diagnostic sampling of aqueous or vitreous for polymerase chain reaction testing can be very helpful to assist in the diagnosis. Systemic antibody testing rarely is indicated. Serial color wide field photographs can be helpful to monitor disease progression. Fluorescein angiography will show hypofluorescence in the areas of necrosis with a characteristic abrupt cut-off of dye in the blood vessels.

Treatment: Antiviral agents (acyclovir, valacyclovir, ganciclovir, valganciclovir, famciclovir, foscarnet) are the mainstay and can be delivered orally, intravenously, and intravitreally, or in combination. Vitrectomy is often required after the acute infection is over, for the management of media opacity and retinal detachment, which commonly develop in the healing phase of the disease.

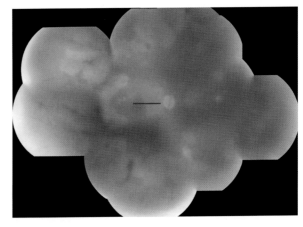

Figure 17.5.1 Color photograph of a patient with acute retinal necrosis at presentation. There is extensive peripheral retinal whitening from necrosis and associated occlusive vasculitis. Red line corresponds to OCT section in Figure 17.5.2.

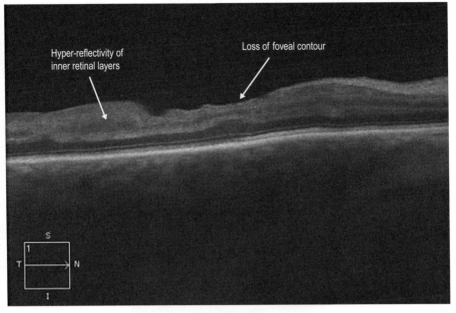

Figure 17.5.2 OCT (corresponding to Figure 17.5.1) shows significant subclinical disease activity that is evident within the macula. Abnormal hyper-reflectivity within the inner retinal layers is a sign of active disease. There is also loss of the normal foveal contour.

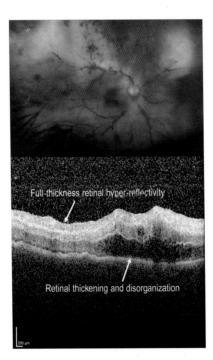

Figure 17.5.3 Widefield image (top) and macular OCT (bottom) of severe, acute varicella zoster virus–associated acute retinal necrosis (ARN) show full-thickness retinal hyper-reflectivity, thickening, and disorganization.

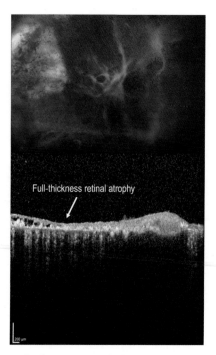

Figure 17.5.4 Widefield image (top) and macular OCT (bottom) 6 weeks following antiviral therapy (corresponding to Figure 17.5.3) show severe, diffuse atrophy involving all retinal layers.

PART 7: Trauma

Section 18: Physical Trauma 204

18.1 Commotio Retinae 204
18.2 Choroidal Rupture and Subretinal Hemorrhage 206
18.3 Valsalva Retinopathy 208

Section 19: Photothermal, Photomechanical, and Photochemical Trauma 210

19.1 Laser Injury (Photothermal and Photomechanical) 210
19.2 Solar Maculopathy 212

18.1 | Commotio Retinae

Introduction: Commotio retinae or Berlin's edema occurs in the setting of nonpenetrating, blunt globe trauma. It may affect any area of the retina and is generally self-limited, but when the macula is involved, visual acuity may be permanently decreased.

Clinical Features: There is retinal whitening caused by damage of the outer retinal layers. The whitening is generally patchy with ill-defined borders and does not follow a vascular distribution (Fig. 18.1.1).

OCT Features: When involving the macula, acutely, there is obscuration of the retinal layers in the involved region with **disruption of the IS–OS/ellipsoid zone and RPE inter-digitation**, sometimes leaving a **cleft of empty, hyporeflective space** under the neurosensory retina (Fig. 18.1.2). There can be a hyper-reflective signal throughout the retinal layers, but this tends to be most pronounced in the **outer layers**. Later, the retina can return to normal in mild cases or there may be permanent loss of outer retina including photoreceptors and the RPE in severe cases (Fig. 18.1.3).

Ancillary Testing: No ancillary testing is generally required.

Treatment: Most cases are self-limiting, but in severe cases where visual damage can occur, no treatment has proven efficacy.

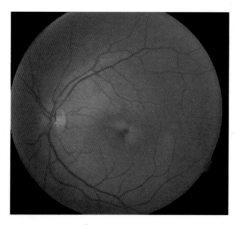

Figure 18.1.1 Color fundus photograph of commotio retinae involving the central macula. Retinal whitening is visible in the affected region.

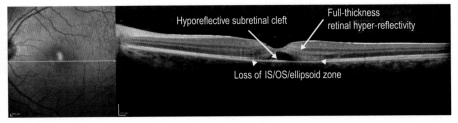

Figure 18.1.2 OCT in the acute setting of commotio retinae shows loss of the IS–OS/ellipsoid zone (between arrowheads) with overlying outer retinal hyper-reflectivity. There is a subretinal cleft of empty, hyporeflective space with surrounding full-thickness retinal hyper-reflectivity.

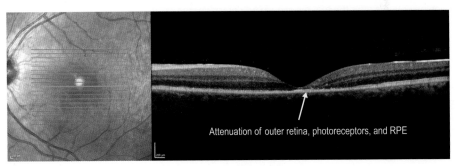

Figure 18.1.3 OCT in the chronic setting of severe commotio retinae shows attenuation of the outer retina, photoreceptors, and retinal pigment epithelium (RPE).

18.2 | Choroidal Rupture and Subretinal Hemorrhage

Introduction: Choroidal ruptures occur after blunt trauma severe enough to cause significant globe compression with subsequent rupture of Bruch's membrane, the retinal pigment epithelium (RPE), and the inner choroid.

Clinical Features: Choroidal ruptures typically occur concentrically to the optic nerve, most commonly temporally and involving the macula (Figs. 18.2.1 and 18.2.2). There is usually associated hemorrhage in the acute setting, which may be located within or underneath the retina. Over time, the hemorrhage will clear, leaving an arc-shaped area of subretinal de-pigmentation with clumps of hyper-pigmentation. Secondary choroidal neovascularization (CNV) can occur months or years after trauma, resulting in further visual loss.

OCT Features: In the acute setting, associated hemorrhage often obscures the presence of a choroidal rupture from view with OCT. As the hemorrhage clears, it becomes more visible and more easily imaged. In the acute or subacute setting, a choroidal rupture appears as an **elevated, nodule-like abnormality spanning Bruch's membrane, the RPE, and inner choroid** (Fig. 18.2.3). With time, the nodular abnormality flattens, leaving a noticeably deformed area that exhibits **negative or reverse shadowing** from focal loss of the RPE (Figs. 18.2.4 and 18.2.5).

Ancillary Testing: Fluorescein angiography and/or indocyanine green angiography can be helpful in identifying the presence of a choroidal rupture site (Fig. 18.2.2) if the diagnosis is in question. Fluorescein angiography can also be helpful to identify an associated CNV, which can develop later in up to 10% of eyes.

Treatment: In the absence of CNV, observation alone is generally advocated. If CNV is present, intravitreal anti-vascular endothelial growth factor therapy is indicated.

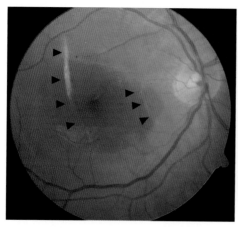

Figure 18.2.1 Color photograph of two separate choroidal rupture sites (arrowheads) and shallow overlying subretinal hemorrhage 2 weeks following blunt trauma. (Courtesy Jeffrey S. Heier, MD.)

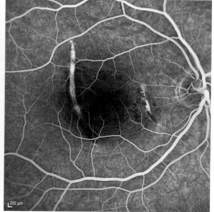

Figure 18.2.2 Fluorescein angiography shows hyper-fluorescence caused by window defects in the location of the two choroidal rupture sites. (Courtesy Jeffrey S. Heier, MD.)

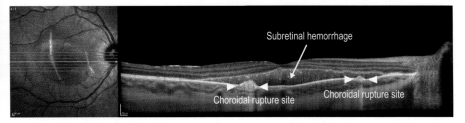

Figure 18.2.3 OCT through two separate choroidal rupture sites two weeks following injury. Overlying subretinal hemorrhage is also present. (Courtesy Jeffrey S. Heier, MD.)

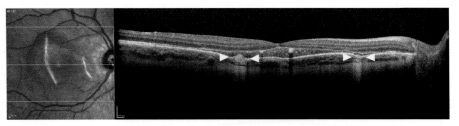

Figure 18.2.4 OCT through the same choroidal rupture sites, 1 month after injury, shows a decrease in size of the nodule-like elevations spanning Bruch's membrane, the retinal pigment epithelium, and inner choroid. (Courtesy Jeffrey S. Heier, MD.)

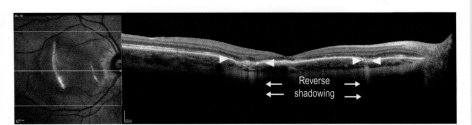

Figure 18.2.5 OCT through the same choroidal rupture sites, 3 months after injury, shows a continued flattening of the choroidal rupture sites. There is negative or reverse shadowing caused by focal loss of the retinal pigment epithelium (between arrowheads). (Courtesy Jeffrey S. Heier, MD.)

Introduction: Valsalva retinopathy results from a sudden increase in intraocular venous pressure caused by forced exhalation against a closed glottis. This leads to rupture of superficial capillaries in predisposed individuals.

Clinical Features: Preretinal hemorrhage accumulates in the sub-internal limiting membrane space, typically overlying the macula (Fig. 18.3.1). With time, the red blood cells layer such that there is a serous component superiorly.

OCT Features: The **superior** serous component forms a **hyporeflective cavity** (Fig. 18.3.2), whereas the **inferior** hemorrhagic component forms a **hyper-reflective cavity** that creates a shadowing artifact of the underlying structures (Fig. 18.3.3). OCT can confirm the specific location of the hemorrhage, such as in the sub-internal limiting membrane space (Fig. 18.3.4). OCT is also helpful to monitor the progression and resolution of hemorrhage over time (Fig. 18.3.5).

Ancillary Testing: Fluorescein angiography and indocyanine green angiography can be used to rule out mimicking lesions such as macro-aneurysms, choroidal neovascularization, or polypoidal choroidal vasculopathy.

Treatment: Observation is appropriate for most cases. Nd:YAG laser membranotomy and surgical evacuation are options in select cases.

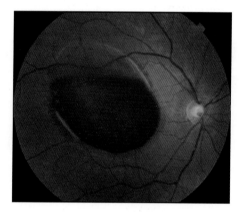

Figure 18.3.1 Color photograph of Valsalva retinopathy with a layered pre-macular hemorrhage. (Modified from Goldman, D. R., & Baumal, C. R. (2014). Natural history of Valsalva retinopathy in an adolescent. *Journal of Pediatric Ophthalmology and Strabismus*, 51(2), 128.)

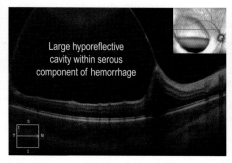

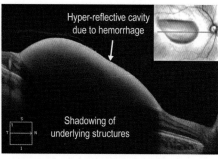

Figure 18.3.2 Horizontal line scan OCT through the superior serous component (corresponding to Figure 18.3.1) shows a large, hyporeflective cavity. (Modified from Goldman, D. R., & Baumal, C. R. (2014). Natural history of Valsalva retinopathy in an adolescent. *Journal of Pediatric Ophthalmology and Strabismus*, 51(2), 128.)

Figure 18.3.3 Horizontal line scan OCT through the inferior hemorrhagic component (corresponding to Fig. 18.3.1) shows a large, hyper-reflective cavity. (Modified from Goldman, D. R., & Baumal, C. R. (2014). Natural history of Valsalva retinopathy in an adolescent. *Journal of Pediatric Ophthalmology and Strabismus*, 51(2), 128.)

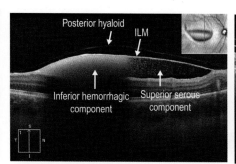

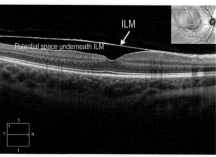

Figure 18.3.4 Vertical line scan OCT shows both the superior serous and inferior hemorrhagic components. Individual red blood cells can be seen disbursed within the serous component. The pre-macular hemorrhage is located underneath the internal limiting membrane (ILM). The posterior hyaloid face can also be seen. (Modified from Goldman, D. R., & Baumal, C. R. (2014). Natural history of Valsalva retinopathy in an adolescent. *Journal of Pediatric Ophthalmology and Strabismus*, 51(2), 128.)

Figure 18.3.5 Upon resolution of the hemorrhage, a potential space underneath the internal limiting membrane (ILM) is still present. (Modified from Goldman, D. R., & Baumal, C. R. (2014). Natural history of Valsalva retinopathy in an adolescent. *Journal of Pediatric Ophthalmology and Strabismus*, 51(2), 128.)

Introduction: Accidental laser injuries to the retina are uncommon but can occur with photothermal injury (typically high-powered handheld laser pointers) and/or photomechanical injury (typically research and military devices).

Clinical Features: The affected region of the retina is typically the central macula. In the acute setting, laser injuries produce a yellow subretinal lesion that can be of varied appearance (Fig. 19.1.1). Within a short time, the affected area becomes pigmented. Eventually, this appearance can resolve leaving more subtle retinal pigment epithelium (RPE) disturbances.

OCT Features: A significant photothermal laser injury causes retinal trauma similar to photocoagulation. On OCT, this is seen as **localized outer retinal, IS–OS/ellipsoid zone, and RPE disruption** in the acute setting (Figs. 19.1.2 and 19.1.3). At the site of injury, subretinal fluid may be present under the retina. The inner retina may also be affected, but usually less so than the inner retina (Fig. 19.1.4). With mild exposure, the findings may be very subtle (Fig. 19.1.5). The abnormalities tend to **fade quickly**, in most cases over weeks to months (Figs. 19.1.6 and 19.1.7).

Ancillary Testing: Fluorescein angiography can be helpful to evaluate for the presence of any associated choroidal neovascularization.

Treatment: As these injuries are very rare, no therapy has been proven to have definite efficacy, although oral corticosteroids have been used in the acute setting.

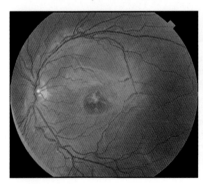

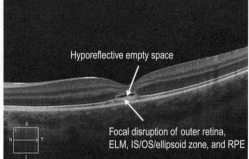

Figure 19.1.1 Color photograph shows yellow subretinal deposits in a splotchy pattern within the central macula. This patient was exposed to a high-powered handheld class 3B laser pointer.

Figure 19.1.2 OCT (corresponding to Figure 19.1.1) shows focal disruption of the outer retina, external limiting membrane (ELM), IS–OS/ellipsoid zone, and retinal pigment epithelium (RPE) underlying the fovea. There is also a thin hyporeflective empty space above the focal disruption.

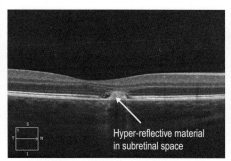

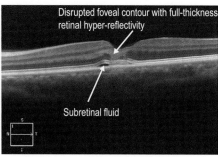

Figure 19.1.3 OCT of a different accidental high-powered laser pointer injury also shows focal disruption of the outer retina, external limiting membrane (ELM), IS–OS/ellipsoid zone, and retinal pigment epithelium (RPE) with a collection of hyper-reflective material under the retina.

Figure 19.1.4 OCT of an accidental military defense laser injury shows an abnormal hyper-reflective signal involving the full thickness of the retina within the fovea. There is also a tiny pocket of subretinal fluid adjacent to the central abnormality.

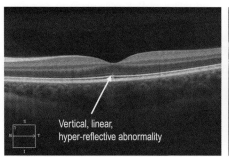

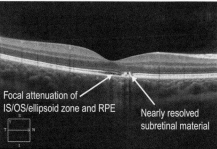

Figure 19.1.5 OCT of the fellow eye of the patient in Figure 19.1.2 shows a subtle abnormality caused by limited exposure of this eye to the laser beam. There is a vertical, linear, hyper-reflective abnormality underneath the center of the fovea that spans from the retinal pigment epithelium (RPE) to the external limiting membrane (ELM).

Figure 19.1.6 One month following the injury (see Figure 19.1.3), OCT shows near resolution of the focal outer retinal disruption and subretinal material. The IS–OS/ellipsoid zone and retinal pigment epithelium (RPE) are still somewhat attenuated underneath the fovea.

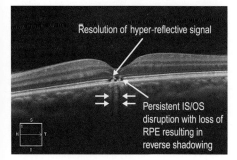

Figure 19.1.7 One month after the injury (see Figure 19.1.4), OCT shows shrinking of the focal outer retinal disruption underneath the fovea and the inner retinal hyper-reflective signal has resolved. *RPE*, retinal pigment epithelium.

19.2 | Solar Maculopathy

Introduction: Accidental retinal light toxicity causes injury to the retina from a photochemical mechanism. This can occur from prolonged exposure to the sun, from a welding arc, and from intraoperative microscope illumination.

Clinical Features: Retinal phototoxicity from the sun or a welding arc appears as a small, round, well-circumscribed, yellow acquired vitelliform-like lesion in the fovea (Fig. 19.2.1). Microscope phototoxicity appears as a broader area that is fairly well circumscribed either in the inferior or superior macula (dependent on tilt of microscope).

OCT Features: Solar and welding arc injuries appear similarly on OCT as a **focal loss of the outer retina** and **IS–OS/ellipsoid layer**, leaving a small **hyporeflective rectangular cavity** or outer retinal hole (Fig. 19.2.2). These lesions can be singular or multifocal with sharply demarcated borders. The inner retina and external limiting membrane (ELM) are spared. OCT defects will typically remain long-term. Microscope light-induced retinal phototoxicity leads to prominent chorioretinal scarring in the region of the injury.

Ancillary Testing: Fluorescein angiography can show a pinpoint window defect centrally in solar retinopathy, but no other imaging modality is as useful as OCT.

Treatment: No treatment is available, but avoidance of additional pathologic light exposure is recommended.

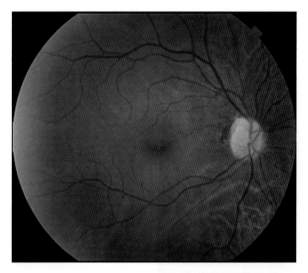

Figure 19.2.1 Color fundus photograph of solar retinal phototoxicity shows a small, central, ovoid light-colored abnormality with a hyper-pigmented rim located in the fovea.

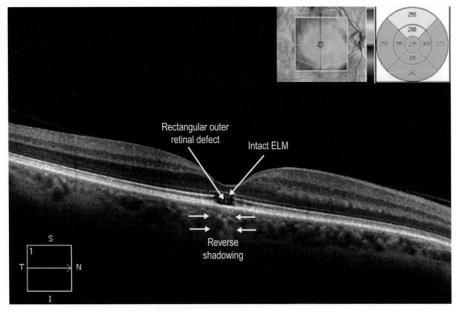

Figure 19.2.2 OCT (corresponding to Figure 19.2.1) shows focal loss of the outer retina including photoreceptors and the IS–OS/ellipsoid layer. In this advanced case, the retinal pigment epithelium (RPE) is also affected, leading to reverse shadowing below (between arrowheads). The overall defect is characteristically rectangle-shaped and the overlying external limiting membrane (ELM) is intact.

PART 8: Tumors

Section 20: Choroidal Tumors 216

    20.1 *Choroidal Nevus* 216
    20.2 *Choroidal Melanoma* 220
    20.3 *Choroidal Hemangioma* 224

Section 21: Retinal Tumors 228

    21.1 *Retinal Capillary Hemangioma* 228
    21.2 *Retinoblastoma* 230

Section 22: Other Tumors 232

    22.1 *Metastatic Choroidal Tumor* 232
    22.2 *Vitreoretinal Lymphoma* 234
    22.3 *Primary Uveal Lymphoma* 238

20.1 Choroidal Nevus

Introduction: Choroidal nevi are common, acquired lesions that are typically discovered during routine funduscopic examination in the absence of symptoms.

Clinical Features: The classic appearance is that of a darkly pigmented, small, flat lesion with well-defined borders (Fig. 20.1.1). Overlying drusen are a common finding suggesting chronicity. Some nevi may have slight elevation (Fig. 20.1.2). Choroidal nevi can occur anywhere in the fundus but are usually seen in the posterior pole. Accumulation of subretinal fluid, minimal growth over time, and alterations in pigmentation can occur in the absence of malignant transformation.

OCT Features: There is **thinning of the choriocapillaris** in the area of the nevus, which appears as a homogeneous **well-defined area of hyper-reflectivity below the retinal pigment epithelium (RPE)** (Figs. 20.1.3 to 20.1.6). The overlying retinal layers are undisturbed. Enhanced depth imaging techniques can help to visualize the more posterior extent of a choroidal nevus (Figs. 20.1.4 and 20.1.6).

Ancillary Testing: B-scan ultrasonography can be used to determine whether the lesion is elevated and measure its dimensions, which aid in distinguishing a choroidal nevus from a choroidal melanoma.

Treatment: No treatment is typically necessary. Serial observation is recommended.

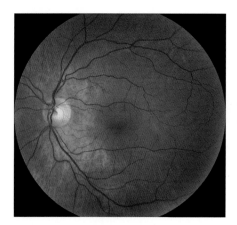

Figure 20.1.1 Color fundus photograph of a small choroidal nevus shows a darkly pigmented, well-circumscribed flat choroidal lesion in the central macula.

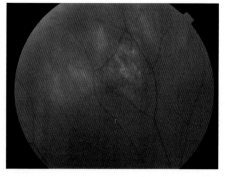

Figure 20.1.2 Color fundus photograph of a minimally elevated nevus shows a darkly pigmented, well-circumscribed choroidal lesion with overlying drusen.

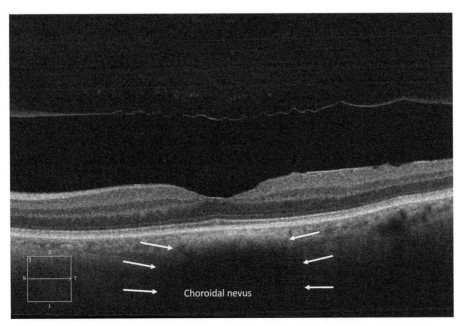

Choroidal nevus

Figure 20.1.3 OCT (corresponding to Figure 20.1.1) shows a small homogeneous, well-defined area of hyper-reflectivity below the retinal pigment epithelium (RPE) that compresses the overlying choriocapillaris in this region, corresponding to the choroidal nevus (arrows).

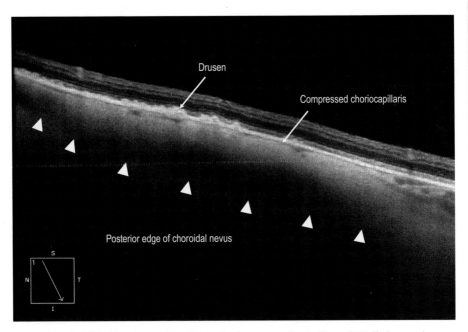

Drusen

Compressed choriocapillaris

Posterior edge of choroidal nevus

Figure 20.1.4 OCT with enhanced depth imaging (corresponding to Figure 20.1.2) shows a larger choroidal nevus with a thin, compressed choriocapillaris and overlying drusen.

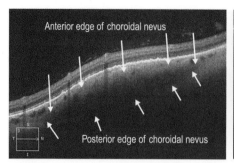

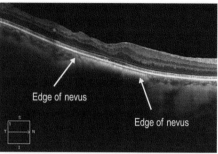

Figure 20.1.5 OCT of another choroidal nevus where the overlying retina has a mild dome-shaped elevation due to the height of the lesion.

Figure 20.1.6 OCT with enhanced depth imaging shows the edges of a flat nevus more clearly. The underlying structures are obscured by shadowing.

Introduction: Choroidal melanoma is the most common primary intraocular malignancy in adults, but it is still quite rare with an incidence of about six per one million people. It most commonly presents in the sixth decade but can affect individuals of any age. In most studied populations, there is a slight predisposition toward males.

Clinical Features: The most common appearance is an abruptly elevated, pigmented, choroidal lesion that enlarges without treatment (Figs. 20.2.1 and 20.2.2). Without documented growth, features such as overlying lipofuscin (orange pigment), associated subretinal fluid, larger size, and proximity to the optic nerve help to differentiate melanoma from benign lesions such as choroidal nevus. On a clinical basis, the diagnosis can be made with greater than 99% accuracy. Biopsy is rarely necessary but can confirm the diagnosis. Radiation retinopathy can often develop after treatment with external radiation (Fig. 20.2.3).

OCT Features: A large homogeneous **hyporeflective, elevated area of choroidal infiltration** is typically seen in association with **overlying subretinal fluid** (Figs. 20.2.4 and 20.2.5). Enhanced depth imaging OCT can assist with the documentation of relatively small melanomas. Older lesions can exhibit cystoid retinal degeneration over the surface of the tumor. More acute lesions tend to show shaggy photoreceptors overlying subretinal fluid. Associated secondary radiation retinopathy can lead to severe **cystoid macular edema** and retinal atrophy (Fig. 20.2.6).

Ancillary Testing: B-scan ultrasonography can be useful in distinguishing choroidal melanoma from benign lesions, such as choroidal nevus. Fluorescein angiography can also be helpful by demonstrating a characteristic internal circulation within the melanoma (Fig. 20.2.2).

Treatment: Radiation therapy (plaque brachytherapy, proton beam, gamma knife) is the most common treatment approach. Enucleation is generally reserved for very large and advanced tumors with poor visual prognosis. Post-radiation retinopathy is common, which can be difficult to treat but is sometimes responsive to focal laser photocoagulation and/or intravitreal anti-vascular endothelial growth factor therapy (Figs. 20.2.7 and 20.2.8).

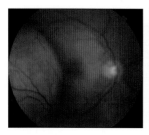

Figure 20.2.1 Color fundus photograph of a large, elevated pigmented choroidal melanoma. The lesion is so elevated that the neighboring macula and optic nerve are out of focus.

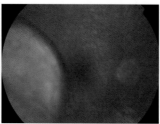

Figure 20.2.2 Late-phase fluorescein angiogram (corresponding to Figure 20.2.1) shows an internal circulation of the choroidal melanoma.

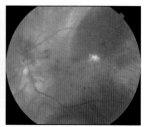

Figure 20.2.3 Color fundus photograph of radiation retinopathy following I-125 plaque brachytherapy for choroidal melanoma. Optic disc edema, intraretinal hemorrhages, cystoid macular edema, and hard exudates are all present.

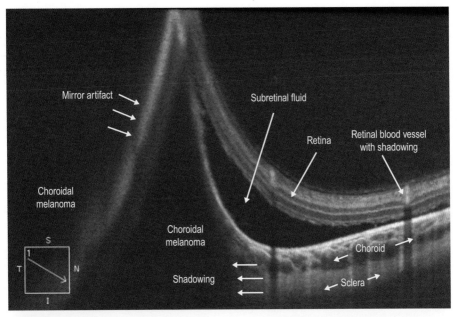

Figure 20.2.4 OCT (corresponding to Figure 20.2.1) shows a large hyporeflective cavity in the choroidal space corresponding to the melanoma with adjacent subretinal fluid. There is mirror artifact overlying the hyporeflective cavity on the left side of the image. There is shadowing underneath the melanoma blocking the choroid and sclera.

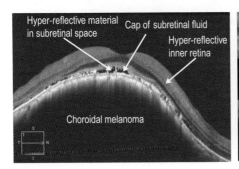

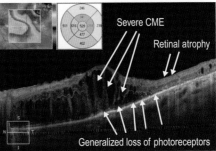

Figure 20.2.5 OCT of a different choroidal melanoma shows a large hyporeflective cavity that has taken over the choroidal space and is elevating the overlying retina. There is a cap of subretinal fluid overlying the lesion and additional hyper-reflective material in the subretinal space, which may represent shed photoreceptors. The inner retina is abnormally hyper-reflective.

Figure 20.2.6 OCT (corresponding to Figure 20.2.3) shows severe cystoid macular edema (CME) due to radiation retinopathy with adjacent retinal atrophy. There is also generalized loss of photoreceptors.

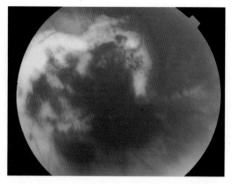

Figure 20.2.7 Color photograph of a regressed choroidal melanoma following distant treatment with plaque brachytherapy.

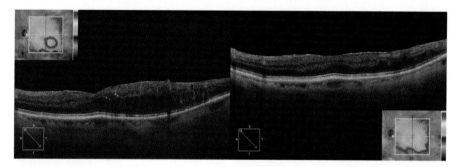

Figure 20.2.8 OCT (corresponding to Figure 20.2.7, macula) shows significant macular edema caused by radiation retinopathy (left). Following serial intravitreal anti-VEGF therapy, the macular edema resolved (right).

Choroidal Hemangioma

Introduction: Choroidal hemangiomas are benign vascular tumors that present in two distinct forms:

▶ Solitary (circumscribed)
▶ Diffuse

The solitary lesions are more common and usually an isolated finding, while the diffuse form is rare and typically associated with Sturge–Weber syndrome.

Clinical Features: Choroidal hemangiomas can be identified as an incidental finding, but they can affect visual acuity if there is associated subretinal fluid or cystic fluid involving the macula. Typical features include a reddish/orange coloration and location in the posterior pole (Fig. 20.3.1). They can be very subtle and easily missed on ophthalmoscopy. Retinal pigment epithelium (RPE) metaplasia on the surface may be present. Occasionally, clinical findings are subtle and only identified on OCT.

OCT Features: There is obscuration of the normal choriocapillaris by a hyporeflective signal and overlying round-shaped retinal elevation (Figs. 20.3.2 and 20.3.3). Overlying subretinal and/or intraretinal fluid may also be present (Fig. 20.3.3), which can involve the macula (Fig. 20.3.4). Occasionally, fluid can occur sub-foveally, even if the tumor is not located within the macula. Enhanced depth imaging techniques can be helpful for better visualization in larger tumors.

Ancillary Testing: Indocyanine green angiography is useful in confirming the diagnosis, particularly in the early phase images 20–30 seconds following injection where prominent hyper-fluorescence of the lesion is noted (Fig. 20.3.5). B-scan ultrasonography can also be helpful.

Treatment: If visual acuity is affected by the presence of subretinal fluid in the macula, photodynamic therapy is the most effective therapy, although various other treatments have been used.

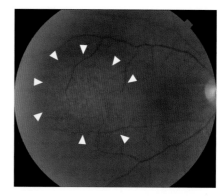

Figure 20.3.1 Color photograph of a clinically evident choroidal hemangioma (arrowheads). There are associated retinal striae, and the foveal reflex is blunted due to the presence of subretinal fluid.

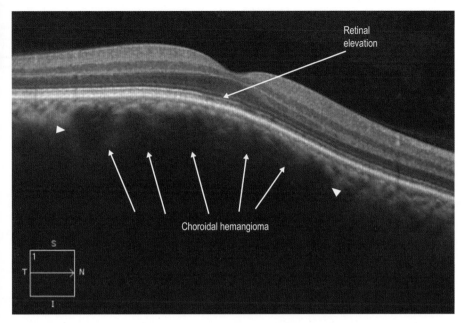

Figure 20.3.2 OCT of a subtle choroidal hemangioma that was not clearly visible clinically. The choriocapillaris is slightly obscured (abnormal hyporeflectivity between arrowheads), and there is elevation of the overlying retina.

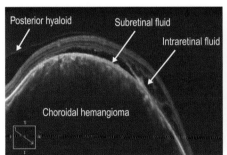

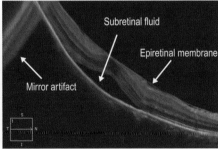

Figure 20.3.3 OCT outside the fovea of a more obvious choroidal hemangioma (corresponding to Figure 20.3.1). The choriocapillaris is completely obscured by the tumor and there is bullous overlying retinal elevation. Subretinal and intraretinal fluid are also present.

Figure 20.3.4 OCT of the fovea (corresponding to Figure 20.3.3) shows the presence of subretinal fluid and a mild epiretinal membrane.

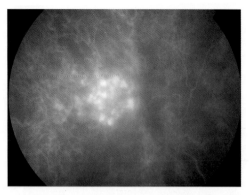

Figure 20.3.5 Indocyanine green angiography at 20 seconds (corresponding to Figure 20.3.1) shows intense early hyper-fluorescence of the choroidal hemangioma, which is a characteristic feature distinguishing this lesion from other choroidal tumors.

Retinal Capillary Hemangioma

Introduction: Retinal capillary hemangiomas (RCH), or hemangioblastomas, are usually seen in association with Von Hippel–Lindau disease, but can also occur sporadically.

Clinical Features: These lesions can affect both the retina and optic nerve. They start out small and can gradually enlarge with the possibility of intraretinal and subretinal exudation that can involve the macula and affect visual acuity. They have characteristic tortuous and dilated feeding and draining arteries and veins (Figs. 21.1.1 and 21.1.2), respectively. Multiple and bilateral lesions are common in the setting of Von Hippel–Lindau disease.

OCT Features: Smaller lesions are seen as a **well-circumscribed** bulbous deformity **obscuring the layers of the retina** (Fig. 21.1.3), whereas larger lesions have a **hyper-reflective inner surface** with deeper structures obscured by shadowing (Fig. 21.1.4). In larger lesions with surrounding exudation, there can be cystoid macular edema (CME) within the retina surrounding the retinal hemangioma (Fig. 21.1.5). Secondarily, there can also be associated intraretinal fluid or even a serous retinal detachment within the macula (Fig. 21.1.6).

Ancillary Testing: Serial color, red-free photos, and ultrasonography can be helpful in tracking changes in lesion size over time. Fluorescein angiography can also be useful in assisting with the diagnosis (Fig. 21.1.2) if it is in question.

Treatment: In general, lesions that are not leaking can be observed. Once peripheral lesions begin to leak, treatment is usually contemplated. Because of the possibility of collateral damage to the optic disc, lesions on the nerve are typically watched until moderate visual loss occurs. Various ablative techniques can be used for therapy, depending on size and location of the lesions, including photodynamic therapy, laser photocoagulation, and cryotherapy.

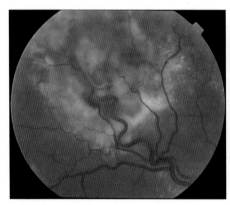

Figure 21.1.1 Color fundus photograph of a retinal capillary hemangioma shows a reddish lesion just superior to the macula with dilated and tortuous feeding vessels. There is surrounding subretinal fluid and exudation present.

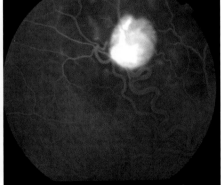

Figure 21.1.2 Late-phase fluorescein angiogram of a retinal capillary hemangioma shows bright hyper-fluorescence of the lesion and highlights the feeding vasculature.

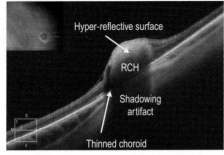

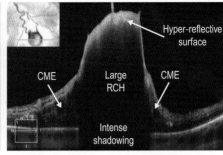

Figure 21.1.3 OCT of a smaller peripheral retinal capillary hemangioma shows a well-circumscribed area of hyper-reflectivity corresponding to the lesion that focally replaces the retina. The underlying choroid appears pinched and thin, although there is significant shadowing artifact. *RCH*, retinal capillary hemangioma

Figure 21.1.4 OCT of a large retinal capillary hemangioma shows hyper-reflectivity of the inner surface. There is dense shadowing of the central and outer portions or the lesion along with underlying retinal and choroidal structures. There is also mild cystoid macular edema (CME) on the edges of the lesion. *RCH*, retinal capillary hemangiomas.

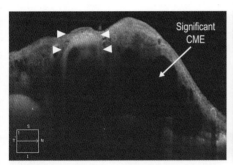

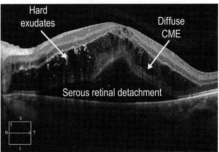

Figure 21.1.5 OCT of a large retinal capillary hemangioma (corresponding to Figure 21.1.1) shows significant hyper-reflectivity of the inner surface of the lesion (between arrowheads). There is also significant surrounding intraretinal fluid or cystoid macular edema (CME).

Figure 21.1.6 OCT of the macula in a patient with a peripheral retinal capillary hemangioma shows significant cystoid macular edema (CME) and a sizeable serous retinal detachment. Hard exudates are also present within the Henle fiber layer (or axonal outer plexiform layer).

Introduction: Retinoblastoma is the most common pediatric intraocular malignancy, representing about 5% of all pediatric malignancies.

Clinical Features: The most common presenting feature is leukocoria, but others signs and symptoms include strabismus, decreased vision, and a painful eye. Characteristic clinical features include a white or yellow-white elevated, fungating, singular or multifocal retinal tumor often with abnormal dilated retinal vasculature feeding the tumor (Fig. 21.2.1). Associated vitreous and subretinal seeding may also be present.

OCT Features: OCT shows involvement of the neurosensory retina, particularly the **photoreceptors** and **outer retina**. Early in tumor growth or along the leading edge of the tumor, these features can be more clearly seen (Fig. 21.2.2). In larger or more advanced tumors, the entire **neurosensory retina can be obscured**, but the underlying **retinal pigment epithelial layer is preserved** (Figs. 21.2.3 and 21.2.4). Retinocytoma is a benign form of retinoblastoma that can be clinically indistinguishable but more differentiated histologically and which carries identical genetic implications. Its OCT features are not distinguishable from retinoblastoma, including internal calcification (Fig. 21.2.5)

Ancillary Testing: Fluorescein angiography may be helpful to differentiate retinoblastoma from other simulating lesions such as Coats disease, toxocariasis, or retinal astrocytoma. Radiography and/or ultrasonography characteristically show internal calcification. Trans-scleral or trans-pars plana biopsy is contraindicated because of the risk of initiating metastasis.

Treatment: Treatment options include intravenous chemotherapy, intra-arterial chemotherapy, cryotherapy, laser photocoagulation, external radiation, and enucleation. The specific treatment is individualized to the unique patient condition.

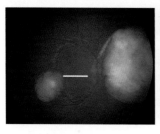

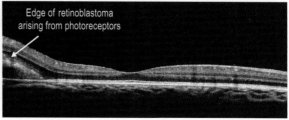

Edge of retinoblastoma arising from photoreceptors

Figure 21.2.1 Color photograph of retinoblastoma in an infant shows two separate lesions involving the posterior pole of differing sizes. Both are round, elevated, and creamy-white. (Courtesy Carol Shields, MD.)

Figure 21.2.2 OCT (corresponding to horizontal line in Figure 21.2.1) shows the edge of the tumor located above the retinal pigment epithelium (RPE) and involving the outer retina. The tumor appears to be arising from the photoreceptor layer. The central fovea is uninvolved. (Courtesy Carol Shields, MD.)

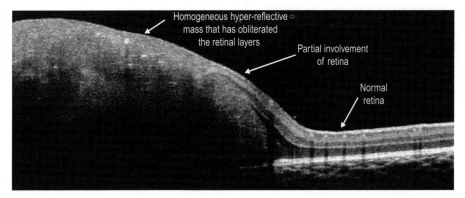

Figure 21.2.3 OCT (corresponding to Figure 21.2.1, horizontal scan through macular lesion) shows a fairly homogeneous hyper-reflective mass that has obliterated the retinal layers completely. The transition to partial involvement of the retina and normal retina can also be seen. (Courtesy Carol Shields, MD.)

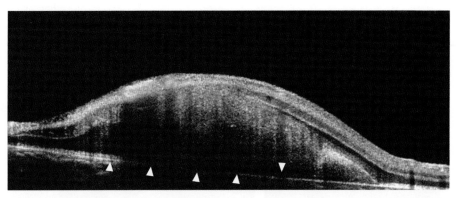

Figure 21.2.4 OCT (corresponding to Figure 21.2.1, vertical scan through macular lesion) illustrates that the underlying retinal pigment epithelium (RPE) layer is intact and not involved (arrowheads). (Courtesy Carol Shields, MD.)

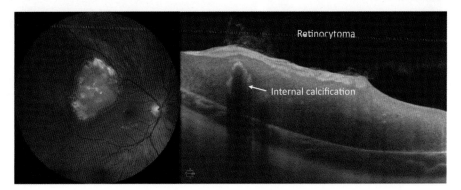

Figure 21.2.5 Color photograph (left) of a retinocytoma shows a whitish, translucent mass. OCT (right) shows a hyper-reflective epiretinal membrane on the surface. The internal appearance is relatively homogeneous with the exception of internal calcification. The areas of calcification have a hyper-reflective rim with internal shadowing and can be seen in both retinoblastoma and retinocytoma. The underlying retinal pigment epithelium (RPE) remains intact.

cube scan, macular, 4–6
cuticular drusen, 42–43
cyclophosphamide, 178, 182
cyclosporine, 174, 178, 182
cystoid macular edema, 96f, 116, 160, 161f
    postoperative, 88, 88f, 89f
cystoid retinal changes, 27, 28f

D

3D scans, 5t
Dalen-Fuch's nodules, 184
diabetic retinopathy
    with macular edema, 126, 127f, 128f, 129f
    non-proliferative, 120, 121f, 122f, 123f, 124f
    proliferative, 130, 131f, 132f, 133f, 134f
disciform scar, 46, 50f
dome-shaped macula, 64, 64f
drusen
    dry AMD, 42–43, 43f, 44f, 45f
    like deposits in RPE, 108, 109f
    overlying, 216, 216f
    shadowing effect of, 20f
dry age-related macular degeneration, 42, 42f,
    43f, 44f, 45f

E

en face images, 6f, 7
en face OCTA images, 8f, 27f
endophthalmitis, Candida albicans endogenous,
    198, 198f, 199f
enhanced depth imaging (EDI), 6
epiretinal membrane, 84, 84f, 85f, 86f, 97f
external limiting membrane, focal loss, 30–31, 31f
exudative retinal detachment, 242

F

famciclovir, 200
floaters, 170, 174
flow deficit, 34–35, 34f
fluorescein angiography
    BRAO, 144, 146f
    choroidal neovascular membrane, 47f, 48f,
        53, 58f
    CRAO, 145f, 148
    macular telangiectasia, 94f
    X-linked juvenile retinoschisis, 116
foscarnet, 200
Fourier domain detection, 2–3
full-thickness macular hole, 78, 78f, 79f
fundus autofluorescence, 162, 163f, 164, 165f
fundus image, 7

G

ganciclovir, 200
ganglion cell complex, 40

H

Harada's disease, 182
Heidelberg Spectralis, 4–7, 5t
hemangioma
    choroidal, 224, 224f, 225f, 226f
    retinal capillary, 228, 228f, 229f
hemeralopia, 166
Hermansky–Pudlak syndrome, 112f, 113, 113f
hydroxychloroquine toxicity, 104, 104f, 105f, 106f
hyper-reflective areas, 10, 148
hyporeflective areas, 10

I

immunoglobulins, 174
indocyanine green angiography, 69f
infliximab, 174, 178, 182
inner segment-outer segment (IS-OS)
        photoreceptor junction, 30–31
interferon alpha-2a, 178
interpretation, 10
    qualitative, 10
    quantitative, 11
intraretinal cysts, 10

K

Kyrieleis plaques, 188, 189f

L

lacquer cracks, 58
lamellar macular hole, 82, 82f, 83f
laser injury, 210, 210f, 211f
line scans, 2, 5t, 6, 6f, 7f, 9, 9f
    optic nerve, 38
lymphoma
    primary uveal, 238, 238f, 239f, 240f
    vitreoretinal, 234, 235f, 236f

M

macula, dome-shaped, 64, 64f
macular capillary dropout, 33f
macular cube scan, 4–6

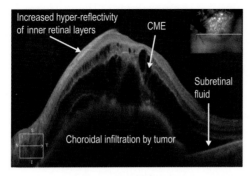

Figure 22.1.3 OCT of a large metastatic choroidal tumor involving the optic nerve and macula shows a hyporeflective elevation of the choroid that is infiltrated by tumor. Overlying this is subretinal fluid and extensive cystoid macular edema (CME). The inner retinal layers are somewhat more hyper-reflective than normal.

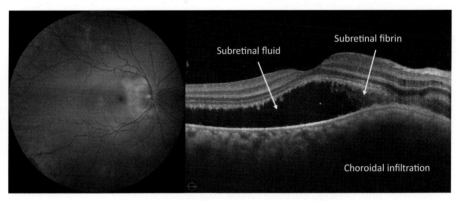

Figure 22.1.4 Color photograph (left) of metastatic breast carcinoma. OCT (right) shows features of choroidal metastases including choroidal infiltration, subretinal fluid, and subretinal fibrin.

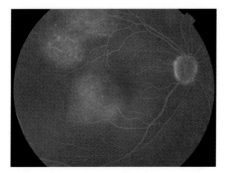

Figure 22.1.5 Fluorescein angiography (corresponding to Figure 22.1.1) shows multiple areas of pinpoint hyper-fluorescence overlying each area of choroidal infiltration. These features are not specific to choroidal metastases.

Vitreoretinal Lymphoma

Introduction: Primary vitreoretinal lymphoma (VRL) is an uncommon form of primary central nervous system lymphoma. Typically it is a malignant B-cell non-Hodgkin lymphoma. Ninety percent of affected patients eventually develop concurrent central nervous system involvement. Historically, the prognosis for survival has been poor, but more recently the prognosis seems to be improving.

Clinical Features: There are no clinical pathognomonic features of VRL, and confirmation of the diagnosis can be difficult, as it typically presents as an unspecified posterior uveitis. In addition to vitreous involvement, lymphoma cells can invade the subretinal and/or subretinal pigment epithelium (RPE) space, leading to characteristic multifocal, dome-shaped, yellowish subretinal deposits. These can be located within the macula but are most striking when located in the retinal periphery (Fig. 22.2.1). Leopard spotting RPE alterations on fundus autofluorescence and fluorescein angiography are typical findings.

OCT Features: The lymphoma cells infiltrate along Bruch's membrane and accumulate as **deposits underneath the RPE**. These deposits appear on OCT as **medium to intense hyper-reflective dome-shaped** sub-RPE elevations of **varying size**. They can be seen both in the macula (Figs. 22.2.2 and 22.2.4) and retinal periphery (Fig. 22.2.3).

Ancillary Testing: Fluorescein angiography and autofluorescence often reveal a leopard spot pattern. A vitrectomy to obtain a diagnostic sample is often necessary to confirm the diagnosis. Pathologic studies employed to confirm the diagnosis include: cytology, immunohistochemistry, flow cytometry, polymerase chain reaction analysis of the immunoglobulin heavy chain gene rearrangement (B-cell lymphoma) and T-cell receptor gene clonality (T-cell lymphoma), IL-10/IL-6 ratio and kappa chain evaluation.

Treatment: Consultation with an oncologist should be undertaken if VRL is suspected. A combination of radiation and systemic chemotherapy is the mainstay of treatment. Intravitreal chemotherapy (methotrexate, rituximab) can be used as adjunctive therapy, particularly when systemic toxicity is an issue.

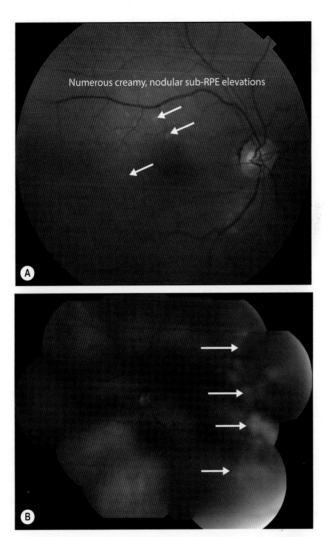

Figure 22.2.1 Color photographs of vitreoretinal lymphoma show numerous creamy, nodular sub-RPE elevations (arrows). Smaller lesions are located in the macula (A), whereas larger lesions are located in the nasal periphery (B).

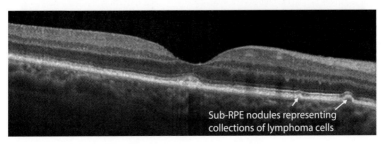

Figure 22.2.2 OCT (corresponding to Figure 22.2.1A) shows small, subretinal pigment epithelium (RPE) nodular elevations that exhibits hyper-reflectivity of medium intensity (arrows). These nodules are believed to be composed of lymphoma cells.

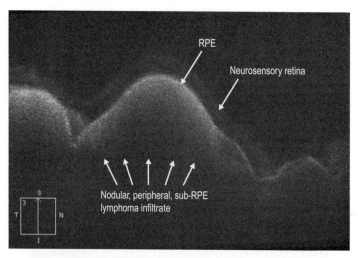

Figure 22.2.3 OCT (corresponding to Figure 22.2.1B) shows numerous large subretinal pigment epithelium (RPE) nodular elevations, which are underneath the neurosensory retina. These larger lesions are intensely hyper-reflective.

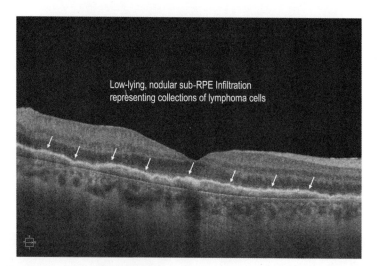

Figure 22.2.4 OCT of a separate vitreoretinal lymphoma case shows a low-lying nodular, but confluent, retinal pigment epithelium (RPE) elevation, which represents diffuse infiltration by lymphoma cells.

Primary Uveal Lymphoma

Introduction: Primary uveal lymphoma is a rare form of (typically B-cell, non-Hodgkin's) intraocular lymphoma that primarily involves the choroid. The disease tends to have an indolent course and is often confused for other masquerading entities, such as scleritis or choroiditis, prior to an accurate diagnosis.

Clinical Features: The most common symptom in affected individuals is decreased visual acuity. Bilateral involvement is common and there is frequently involvement of the surrounding conjunctiva (salmon patch) and orbit. Discrete, yellow-white infiltrates located in the mid to far periphery are present in the vast majority of cases. Diffuse infiltration of the choroid and choroidal folds is sometimes present. Although posterior pole involvement is only present in about half of cases, this location provides the best opportunity for ancillary OCT imaging to aid in the diagnosis.

OCT Features: As the pathology is located beneath the retina, enhanced depth imaging techniques to better visualize the choroid can be helpful. Visualization of choroidal lymphoma on OCT is typified by **extreme thickening/infiltration** and decreased reflectivity **of the choroid** with **loss of typical vascular features** (Figs. 22.3.1 to 22.3.3). **Choroidal folds** with irregular undulations are seen in some cases.

Ancillary Testing: Although biopsy remains the gold standard for diagnosis, B-scan ultrasonography, fluorescein angiography, indocyanine green angiography, and neuroimaging can all be helpful.

Treatment: Observation is done in mild, non-progressive cases with no sight-threatening complications. External beam radiation is quite effective and sufficient therapy for the majority of cases where there is isolated choroidal alone or with orbital involvement (Fig. 22.3.3). Chemo- and immunomodulatory therapy provide adjuvant options for more extensive disease. The majority of cases experience complete remission with treatment.

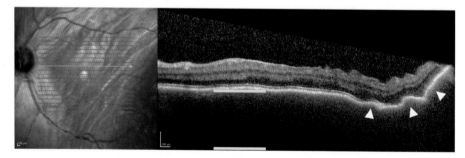

Figure 22.3.1 OCT B-scan of primary choroidal lymphoma exhibits complete obliteration of the choroidal vasculature with diffuse infiltration and thickening of the choroid, spanning the entire lower extent of the imaged region (between yellow bars). The infiltrated region exhibits an upward mechanical effect that causes elevation and irregular folding of the overlying RPE and retinal layers (arrowheads). (Courtesy William J. Harbour, MD.)

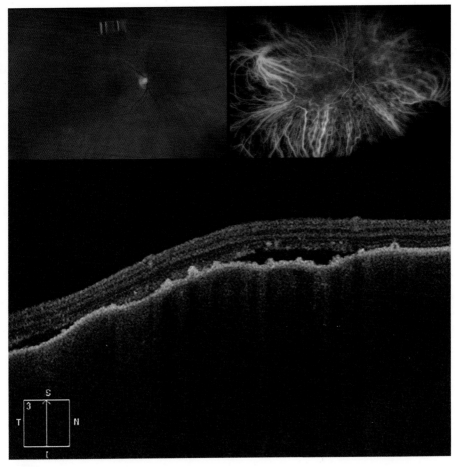

Figure 22.3.2 Color photograph, indocyanine-green angiogram (ICGA), and OCT B-scan of primary choroidal lymphoma involving the posterior pole. Many well-circumscribed yellow-white choroidal infiltrates are apparent in the color photograph with corresponding hypofluorescent lesions on ICGA. OCT shows extreme choroidal thickening with areas of overlying subretinal fluid. (Courtesy Arun D. Singh, MD.)

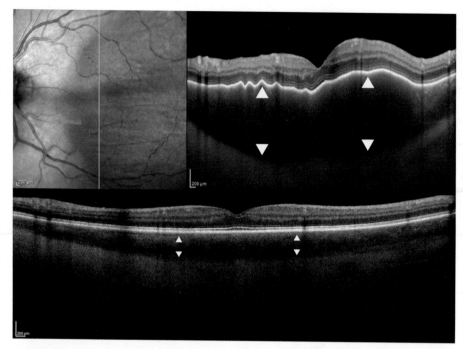

Figure 22.3.3 Infrared image and OCT B-scan of primary choroidal lymphoma at presentation (top). Patient received ultra-low-dose external beam radiation therapy with 4 Gy of radiation delivered over two sessions with complete regression of the lesion (bottom). Diffuse choroidal infiltration with thickening and loss of the choroidal vasculature is noted prior to treatment, followed by resumption of normal choroidal thickness and vasculature after treatment (between arrowheads). (From Yang X, Dalvin LA, Lim LS, Mashayekhi A, Shields JA, Shields CL. Ultra-low-dose (boom boom) radiotherapy for choroidal lymphoma in three consecutive cases. *Eur J Ophthalmology*. 2019, doi: 10.1177/1120672119888985; Images courtesy Carol L. Shields, MD.)

PART 9: Peripheral Retinal Abnormalities

Section 23: Retinal Detachment 242

23.1 Retinal Detachment 242
Omar Abu-Qamar

Section 24: Retinoschisis 244

24.1 Retinoschisis 244
Omar Abu-Qamar

Section 25: Peripheral Lattice Degeneration...248

25.1 Peripheral Lattice Degeneration 248
Omar Abu-Qamar

23.1 | Retinal Detachment

Introduction: Retinal detachment (RD) is a separation of the neurosensory retina from the underlying retinal pigment epithelium. There are three different forms of RDs:

▸ Rhegmatogenous
▸ Exudative
▸ Tractional

Some eyes present with a combination of these three. Tractional and exudative detachments are discussed in greater detail in the chapters associated with their underlying pathologies. Rhegmatogenous RD is more common in men, particularly those between 40 and 70 years of age. Risk factors for rhegmatogenous RD include prior cataract surgery, myopia, trauma, peripheral lattice degeneration, a family history of rhegmatogenous RD, retinal tears, and other intraocular surgery. Tractional RDs occur most commonly in the setting of fibrous membranes in the vitreous, secondary to diseases such as proliferative diabetic retinopathy, retinopathy of prematurity, sickle cell retinopathy, trauma, or proliferative vitreoretinopathy. Exudative RDs occur secondary to neoplastic or inflammatory processes, central serous chorioretinopathy, or uveal effusion syndrome.

Clinical Features: Patients with rhegmatogenous RD present with painless unilateral decrease in vision or visual field with flashes and floaters. Most eyes have a posterior vitreous detachment. Examination reveals elevation of the retina, with a corrugated appearance and generally clear subretinal fluid that does not shift with position. The pathognomonic sign of a rhegmatogenous RD is the presence of one or more retinal tears or full-thickness retinal breaks (Fig. 23.1.1).

Exudative RDs are serous, with a smooth surface and shifting subretinal fluid. Other signs may be seen depending on the etiology.

Tractional RDs show preretinal proliferation with traction on the retinal surface and elevated, taut retina.

OCT Features: OCT of RD shows **elevation of the neurosensory retina** from the underlying retinal pigment epithelium (RPE) (Figs. 23.1.2 and 23.1.3). No splitting of retinal layers is seen except in the setting of combined retinoschisis-rhegmatogenous RD. Occasionally, RDs, especially chronic RDs, may be associated with **cystic changes** within the retina. The subretinal fluid in rhegmatogenous RDs is usually **clear** and **hyporeflective**.

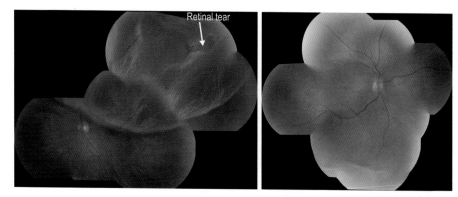

Figure 23.1.1 Color photograph shows a rhegmatogenous retinal detachment with a retinal tear. Note the corrugated, transparent retinal surface. The second photograph shows a serous retinal detachment.

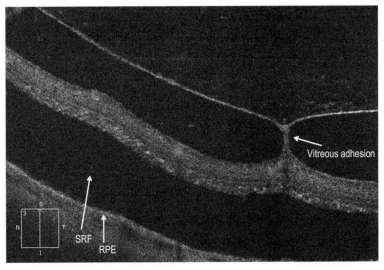

Figure 23.1.2 OCT scan through a retinal detachment shows separation of the neurosensory retina from the hyper-reflective underlying retinal pigment epithelium (RPE). Subretinal fluid (SRF) can be seen. Note the site of vitreous attachment on the retina.

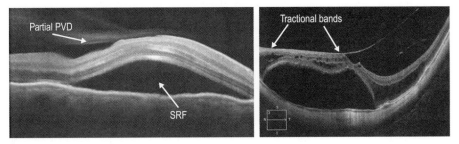

Figure 23.1.3 OCT scan through a serous retinal detachment on the left and a tractional detachment on the right. Note the smooth surface of the serous detachment and the preretinal fibrous tractional bands and hyaloidal thickening in the tractional retinal detachment. *PVD*, posterior vitreous detachment

Tractional RDs show **hyper-reflective bands** that attach to the inner retina and cause retinal elevation.

Serous RDs are occasionally associated with **turbid subretinal fluid** that is hyper-reflective.

Ancillary Testing: The diagnosis of rhegmatogenous RD is made on clinical examination. Tractional and serous RDs may need additional testing based on the underlying pathophysiology. B-scan ultrasonography is critical in the setting of cloudy media.

Management: Rhegmatogenous RD usually requires surgical intervention, with pneumatic retinopexy, vitrectomy surgery, scleral buckling surgery, or a combination of both. Laser demarcation is an option in peripheral rhegmatogenous RD.

The management of tractional and serous RDs depends on their underlying etiology and the location of the detachment in relation to the macula.

24.1 Retinoschisis

Introduction: Retinoschisis is defined as splitting of the retinal layers. In the peripheral retina, it occurs in a senile (more common) and a juvenile X-linked form. Traction on the macula can also induce macular retinoschisis. This is most commonly seen in highly myopic individuals but can rarely occur secondary to an epiretinal membrane or in an otherwise normal eye. Senile retinoschisis is estimated to occur in 4% of eyes of normal individuals. There is no gender preponderance. Most are stable and chronic, but some (around 1%) may progress to retinal detachment after developing inner and outer retinal holes or just outer retinal holes.

Juvenile retinoschisis is a rare and usually X-linked condition that occurs in men. It is congenital, but its manifestations may not be apparent until later in life.

Clinical Presentation: Senile retinoschisis is usually bilateral, with a smooth, domed appearance and most commonly develops inferotemporally (Fig. 24.1.1). There may be non-inflammatory sheathing of retinal blood vessels and retinal "snowflakes" seen over the inner wall of the schisis cavity. An absolute scotoma is seen on visual field testing, in contrast to the relative scotoma seen in acute rhegmatogenous retinal detachment. Both inner and outer retinal breaks may be seen, but rarely in conjunction. Unlike a retinal detachment, no demarcation line is seen, unless the schisis progresses into a combined detachment.

Patients with juvenile X-linked retinoschisis demonstrate decreased vision associated with macular schisis. More severe loss of vision can occur as a result of recurrent vitreous hemorrhage or combined schisis-rhegmatogenous retinal detachment.

OCT Features: Line scans through the area of retinoschisis show a **splitting** of the neurosensory retina, with the split between the inner and outer retinal layers, in contrast to a retinal detachment where the separation is between the retinal pigment epithelium and the neurosensory retina (Figs. 24.1.2 and 24.1.3). **Hyporeflective spaces** in the nerve fiber layer may represent cystic degeneration.

In juvenile retinoschisis, OCT demonstrates foveal cystic alterations primarily in the outer retinal layers, but eventually the inner retina can be involved as well (Figs. 24.1.4 and 24.1.5). OCT of the peripheral schisis shows cleavage in the retinal tissue, with bridging retinal elements seen traversing the schisis cavity.

Ancillary Testing: None is needed. Occasionally, visual field testing may be obtained to confirm the presence of an absolute scotoma.

Treatment: Surgery or laser demarcation is indicated only for eyes that develop a concomitant rhegmatogenous retinal detachment in senile retinoschisis.

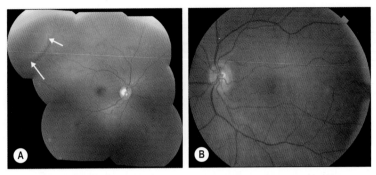

Figure 24.1.1 (A) Fundus photograph of a patient with peripheral retinoschisis (arrows). (B) Fundus photograph of a patient with macular schisis. Note the characteristic cartwheel appearance of the macula.

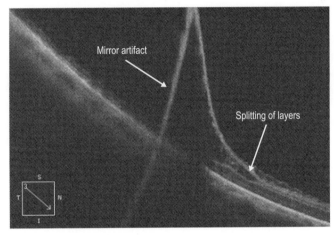

Figure 24.1.2 OCT scan through an area of retinoschisis. Note that the inner and outer retinal layers are separated. Also note the artifactual line seen because the retinoschisis crosses the zero delay line of the OCT scanner.

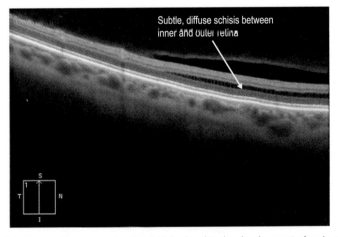

Figure 24.1.3 OCT scan through early retinoschisis showing the development of early cystic changes.

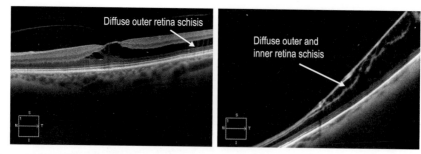

Figure 24.1.4 OCT scans through an area of juvenile retinoschisis. There is schisis with cystic changes at the fovea. There is also peripheral retinoschisis with bands of tissue crossing the schisis cavity.

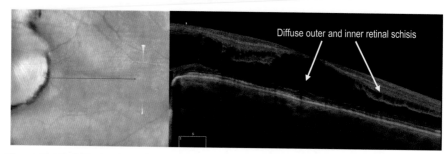

Figure 24.1.5 OCT scan through an area of schisis caused by traction in an eye with retinopathy of prematurity.

25.1 | Peripheral Lattice Degeneration

Introduction: Lattice degeneration is a common finding in the peripheral retina. It is characterized by localized retinal thinning with overlying premature vitreous syneresis and traction. This commonly results in atrophic holes; retinal tears and subsequent retinal detachment are much more uncommon. This condition is estimated to occur in about 8% of the general population and is more common in moderately myopic individuals. Approximately 40% of eyes with retinal detachment have lattice degeneration.

Clinical Findings: The vast majority of affected patients are asymptomatic, with lattice being noted as an incidental finding on a dilated retinal examination. Some patients may complain of photopsias and floaters. Typical lattice consists of sharply demarcated spindle-shaped areas of retinal thinning usually located in the retinal periphery between the equator of the retina and the posterior border of the vitreous base (Fig. 25.1.1). Lattice degeneration occurs more frequently temporally and superiorly in the retina. The retina may be thinned and atrophic. Atrophic holes are the most commonly seen type of retinal break, which typically remain stable, and are rarely associated with retinal detachment. Occasionally, vitreous traction over lattice can cause formation of horseshoe retinal tears, which may result in retinal detachment.

OCT Features: **Posterior vitreous separation** may be noted over the area of the lattice. Alternatively, **adherence of the vitreous** over the area of the lattice with separation of vitreous anterior and posterior to the lattice may cause a **U-shaped appearance** to the vitreous (Fig. 25.1.2). This area of U-shaped traction may be associated with **focal retinal detachment** with **hyper-reflective areas** within the retina representing disruption of normal cell structure or pigment migration. **Retinal thinning** may also be seen in the area of lattice with the inner retina most severely affected. Areas of **atrophic holes** may be seen within these areas of lattice. **Vitreous membranes** and **cellular aggregates** may also be seen in the vitreous of eyes with lattice degeneration (Figs. 25.1.3 and 25.1.4).

Ancillary Testing: Lattice degeneration is best seen with indirect ophthalmoscopy. No ancillary testing is usually needed.

Treatment: Lattice degeneration is usually managed with observation. Based on the low incidence of retinal detachment associated with lattice degeneration and atrophic holes, there is little benefit and even potential harm in prophylactic treatment of lattice and atrophic holes in lattice. However, acute symptomatic retinal holes and tears are treated with prophylactic laser to prevent progression to a retinal detachment.

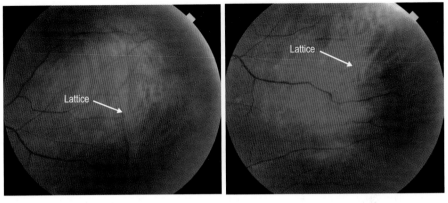

Figure 25.1.1 Fundus photographs showing lattice degeneration in the mid-peripheral retina (arrows).

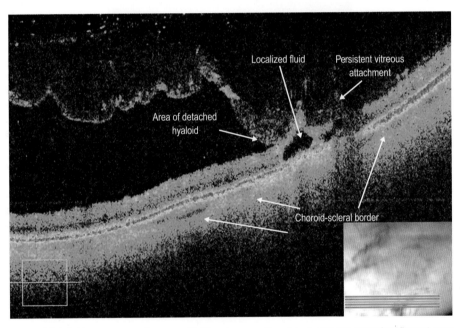

Figure 25.1.2 Line scan over the area of lattice degeneration shows vitreous strongly adherent over the area of the lattice (between arrows) and detached anterior to the lattice. There is traction with a focal tractional detachment over the area of lattice. There is thinning of the retina, especially the inner retina. Also note the thinned choroid characteristic of myopia.

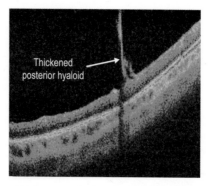

Figure 25.1.3 A fibrous band/thickened posterior hyaloid face is seen exerting traction over the area of lattice.

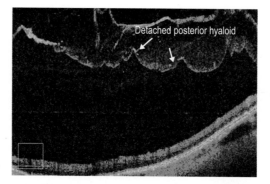

Figure 25.1.4 Debris and cellular aggregates are seen within the vitreous (arrows).

Introduction: Choroidal metastatic lesions are the most common malignant intraocular tumors in adults. The most common primary sites are breast and lung.

Clinical Features: These lesions are typically creamy, yellow, and elevated. They tend to be bilateral and can also be multifocal (Fig. 22.1.1). Associated serous retinal detachments can cause decreased visual acuity when involving the macula. A history of primary malignancy is helpful in confirming the diagnosis.

OCT Features: There is elevation of the choroid in the location of the tumor, which can have overlying subretinal fluid (Fig. 22.1.2). Other associated features include cystoid intraretinal fluid overlying the tumor (Fig. 22.1.3) and subretinal fibrin (Fig. 22.1.4).

Ancillary Testing: B-scan ultrasonography is particularly helpful in providing supportive evidence for the diagnosis with metastatic choroidal lesions typically displaying moderate to high internal reflectivity. Fluorescein angiography is not particularly helpful in differentiating metastatic from primary choroidal tumors (Fig. 22.1.5).

Treatment: The need for local treatment depends on the type and extent of metastatic lesions, as many respond adequately to systemic chemotherapy. Any of the various external radiation modalities can be used as adjunctive therapy, when necessary.

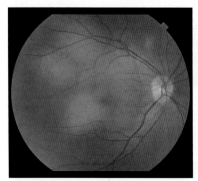

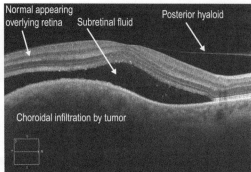

Figure 22.1.1 Color fundus photograph shows numerous creamy, yellowish, circular, minimally elevated choroidal tumors within the posterior pole in a patient with pulmonary metastases.

Figure 22.1.2 OCT (corresponding to Figure 22.1.1) shows a hill-like elevation of the choroid due to infiltration by the tumor with mild obscuration of the choriocapillaris. There is overlying subretinal fluid.

Index

Page numbers followed by 'f' indicate figures, 't' indicate tables.

A

A-scan, 2
acute retinal necrosis syndrome, 200, 200f, 201f, 202f
acute syphilitic posterior placoid chorioretinitis, 196, 196f, 197f
acyclovir, 200
aflibercept, 140
age-related macular degeneration
    dry, 42, 42f, 43f, 44f, 45f
    wet, 46, 47f, 48f, 49f, 50f, 51f, 52f, 53f, 54f
albinism, oculocutaneous, 112, 112f, 113f
AMD. See age-related macular degeneration
artifacts, 12–16
    blink, 14–15, 17f
    mirror, 12, 13f
    misalignment, 12–13, 14f
    motion, 15–16, 17f
    out of range error, 16, 18f
    projection, 18, 21f
    segmentation, 18, 22f
    software breakdown, 13–14, 15f, 16f
    vignetting, 12, 13f
azathioprine, 174, 178, 182

B

B-scan. See line scans
Berlin's edema, 204, 204f, 205f
Best disease, 164, 164f, 165f
bevacizumab, 140
Bioptogen SD-OCT, 5t
birdshot chorioretinopathy, 174, 175f, 176f, 177f
blink artifact, 14–15, 17f
box scans, 5t
branch retinal artery obstruction, 144, 144f, 145f, 146f
branch retinal vein obstruction, 136, 136f, 137f, 138f
BRAO. See branch retinal artery obstruction
Bruch's membrane, 29, 42–43, 68–70
    choroidal neovascular membrane, 58
bull's eye maculopathy, 104, 104f, 106f, 162f

C

C-scans, 6f, 7
Candida albicans endogenous endophthalmitis, 198, 198f, 199f
Canon HS-100, 5t
capillary dropout, 33–34, 33f
central retinal artery obstruction, 148, 148f, 149f, 150f
central retinal vein obstruction, 140, 141f, 142f
central serous chorioretinopathy, 46–47, 65, 68–70, 69f, 100, 100f, 101f, 102f
Chediak–Higashi syndrome, 112f, 113, 113f
cherry-red spot, 148, 148f
chlorambucil, 182
choriocapillaris flow deficits, 34, 34f
chorioretinal atrophy, 58
chorioretinitis
    acute syphilitic posterior placoid, 196, 196f, 197f
    toxoplasmic, 188, 188f, 189f, 190f
    tubercular, 192, 192f, 193f
chorioretinopathy
    birdshot, 174, 175f, 176f, 177f
    central serous, 46–47, 65, 68–70, 69f, 100, 100f, 101f, 102f
choroidal hemangioma, 224, 224f, 225f, 226f
choroidal melanoma, 220, 220f, 221f, 222f
choroidal neovascular membrane, myopic, 58, 58f, 59f, 60f, 61f
choroidal neovascularization, 31–33, 164
choroidal nevus, 216, 216f, 217f, 218f
choroidal rupture, 206, 206f, 207f
choroiditis
    multifocal, 170, 170f, 171f, 172f
    serpiginous, 178, 179f, 180f
cilioretinal artery obstruction, 152, 152f, 153f
Cirrus HD-OCT, 38
commotio retinae, 204, 204f, 205f
cone dystrophy, 166, 166f, 167f
cone–rod retinitis pigmentosa, 166
corticosteroids, 140, 210
cotton wool spots, 120, 121f, 136f, 137f, 154, 157f
CRAO. See central retinal artery obstruction
cross-line scans, 5t, 6

macular degeneration, age-related. *See* age-related macular degeneration
macular edema
    CRVO, 140
    with non-proliferative diabetic retinopathy, 126, 127f, 128f, 129f
    postoperative cystoid, 88, 88f, 89f
macular hole, full-thickness, 78, 78f, 79f
macular maps, 7, 7f
macular neovascularization, 31–33, 32f
macular schisis, myopic, 62, 62f, 63f
macular telangiectasia, 90
    type 1, 90f, 91f
    type 2, 90f, 92f, 93f, 94f
maps
    macular, 7, 7f
    nerve fiber layer, 7f, 8
    topographical, 7f, 8
melanoma, choroidal, 220, 220f, 221f, 222f
mesh scans, 5t, 6
metamorphopsia, 74
metastatic choroidal tumor, 232, 232f, 233f
methotrexate, 174
microaneurysms, 35, 35f
mirror artifact, 12, 13f
misalignment, 12–13, 14f
MNV. *See* macular neovascularization
motion artifact, 15–17, 17f, 19f
Müller cells, 62
multifocal choroiditis, 170, 170f, 171f, 172f
Mycobacterium tuberculosis,192, 192f, 193f, 194f
mycophenolate mofetil, 174
myopic choroidal neovascular membrane, 58, 58f, 59f, 60f, 61f
myopic macular schisis, 62, 62f, 63f
myopic tractional retinal detachment, 66, 66f

N

neovascularization of the optic disc, 131f, 133f, 134f
nerve fiber layer. *See* retinal nerve fiber layer
Nidek OCT RS-3000, 5t
non-proliferative diabetic retinopathy, 120, 121f, 122f, 123f, 124f
    with macular edema, 126, 127f, 128f, 129f
normal vasculature, 26
NVD. *See* neovascularization of the optic disc
nyctalopia, 160, 174

O

OCT. *See* optical coherence tomography
OCTA. *See* optical coherence tomography angiography

oculocutaneous albinism, 112, 112f, 113f
ophthalmia, sympathetic, 184, 184f, 185f
optic atrophy, 174
optic disc
    edema, 170f
    neovascularization, 131f, 133f, 134f
optic nerve
    circle scans, 38
    ganglion cell complex, 40
    line scans, 38
    morphology, 39–40
    scan patterns, 38, 39f
    volume scans, 38
optical coherence tomography
    interpretation, 10
    scan patterns and output, 5t
    scanning principles, 2
optical coherence tomography angiography
    motion artifact, 16–17, 19f
    projection artifact, 18, 21f
    qualitative interpretation, 10
    quantitative interpretation, 11
    scan patterns and output, 8–9, 8f
    scanning principles, 3
    segmentation artifact, 18, 22f
    shadowing, 17–18, 20f
    vascular pathology on, 31–33
optical frequency domain OCT. *See* swept source OCT
out of range error, 16, 18f

P

pachychoroid neovasculopathy, 68
pachychoroid pigment epitheliopathy, 68–70, 70f
pachychoroid syndrome, 68, 68f, 69f, 70f, 71f, 72f
pachydrusen, 68, 70, 72f
pachyvessels, 68–70, 69f
paracentral acute middle maculopathy, 154, 155f, 156f, 157f
pars planitis, 97f
pattern dystrophy, 108, 108f, 109f, 110f
perfluorocarbon, subretinal, 114, 114f, 115f
peripheral lattice degeneration, 248, 249f, 250f
photomechanical laser injury, 210, 210f, 211f
photopsia, 170, 174
photothermal laser injury, 210, 210f, 211f
pisciform flecks, 162, 162f
polypoidal choroidal vasculopathy, 46, 53f, 68–70, 71f
posterior scleritis, 186, 186f, 187f
postoperative cystoid macular edema, 88, 88f, 89f
preretinal hemorrhage, 208, 208f

primary uveal lymphoma, 238, 238*f*, 239*f*, 240*f*
projection artifact, 18, 21*f*
proliferative diabetic retinopathy, 130, 131*f*,
    132*f*, 133*f*, 134*f*

Q

qualitative evaluation, 10

R

radial scans, 4, 5*t*
ranibizumab, 140
raster scans, 4–6
registration, 10
rendered fundus image, 7
retina
    acute retinal necrosis syndrome, 200, 200*f*,
        201*f*, 202*f*
    angiomatous proliferation, 51*f*
    atrophy, 163*f*
    cystic changes, 27, 28*f*
    focal loss of external limiting membrane,
        30–31, 31*f*
    myopic tractional detachment, 66, 66*f*
    normal anatomy, 24, 24*f*
    subretinal fluid, 27–29, 28*f*
retinal angiomatosis proliferation, 46, 51*f*, 52*f*
retinal artery obstruction
    branch, 144, 144*f*, 145*f*, 146*f*
    central, 148, 148*f*, 149*f*, 150*f*
retinal capillary hemangioma, 228, 228*f*, 229*f*
retinal detachment, 242, 242*f*, 243*f*
    exudative, 242
    myopic tractional, 66, 66*f*
    retinal pigment epithelium, 29, 30*f*, 46–47,
        48*f*, 49*f*, 51*f*, 52*f*, 54*f*
    rhegmatogenous, 242–243, 242*f*
    tractional, 130, 132*f*, 242–243, 243*f*
retinal neovascularization, 33
retinal nerve fiber layer, 38–40
    maps, 7*f*, 8
    thickness, 38–39, 39*f*
retinal pigment epithelium, 10, 24, 42, 108
    atrophy, 29–30, 30*f*, 78–80, 164
    detachment, 29, 30*f*, 46–47, 48*f*, 49*f*, 51*f*,
        52*f*, 54*f*
    posterior staphyloma, 56*f*
    tear, 46, 49*f*, 50*f*
retinal striae, 84*f*
retinal vein obstruction
    branch, 136, 136*f*, 137*f*, 138*f*
    central, 140, 141*f*, 142*f*
retinitis pigmentosa, 160, 160*f*, 161*f*
    cone–rod, 166

retinoblastoma, 230, 230*f*, 231*f*
retinopathy
    hydroxychloroquine-induced, 104, 104*f*, 105*f*,
        106*f*
    Valsalva, 208, 208*f*, 209*f*
retinoschisis, 244, 245*f*, 246*f*
    X-linked juvenile, 116, 116*f*, 117*f*, 118*f*
reverse shadowing, 10, 42–43, 44*f*
rhegmatogenous retinal detachment, 242–243,
    242*f*
RT-Vue, 4, 5*t*

S

sampling error, 10
sarcoid anterior uveitis, 97*f*
sarcoid posterior uveitis, 96*f*, 98*f*
scan patterns, 5*t*
    optic nerve, 38
scanning speed, 2–3
scleritis, posterior, 186, 186*f*, 187*f*
SCP. *See* superficial capillary plexus
segmentation artifact, 18, 22*f*
sensitivity roll-off, 24
serpiginous choroiditis, 178, 179*f*, 180*f*
shadowing, 10
    OCTA angiography, 17–18, 20*f*
    reverse, 10, 42–43, 44*f*
software breakdown, 13–14, 15*f*, 16*f*
solar maculopathy, 212, 212*f*, 213*f*
spectral domain detection, 2
staphyloma, posterior, 56, 56*f*, 57*f*
Stargardt disease, 162, 162*f*, 163*f*
subretinal fluid, 27–29, 28*f*, 78–80, 137*f*
    turbidity, 28–29, 29*f*
subretinal hemorrhage, 206, 206*f*, 207*f*
summed voxel projection, 7
superficial capillary plexus, 8*f*, 9*f*, 27*f*, 33*f*, 35*f*
swept source OCT, 2–3, 24
sympathetic ophthalmia, 184, 184*f*, 185*f*

T

telangiectasia, macular, 90
time domain detection, 2
Topcon 3D OCT, 4–6, 5*t*
topographical maps, 7*f*, 8
toxoplasmic chorioretinitis, 188, 188*f*, 189*f*, 190*f*
tractional retinal detachment, 130, 132*f*, 242–
    243, 243*f*
trauma
    choroidal rupture, 206, 206*f*, 207*f*
    commotio retinae, 204, 204*f*, 205*f*
    laser injury, 210, 210*f*, 211*f*
    retinal light toxicity, 212

Index

subretinal hemorrhage, 206, 206f, 207f
  Valsalva retinopathy, 208, 208f, 209f
tuberculosis, 192, 192f, 193f, 194f
tumors
  choroidal hemangioma, 224, 224f, 225f, 226f
  choroidal melanoma, 220, 220f, 221f, 222f
  choroidal nevus, 216, 216f, 217f, 218f
  metastatic choroidal, 232, 232f, 233f
  retinal capillary hemangioma, 228, 228f, 229f
  retinoblastoma, 230, 230f, 231f
  vitreoretinal lymphoma, 234, 235f, 236f

U

uveitis, 96, 97f, 98f
  sarcoid anterior, 97f
  sarcoid posterior, 96f, 98f

V

valacyclovir, 200
valganciclovir, 200
Valsalva retinopathy, 208, 208f, 209f
vignetting, 12, 13f
vitreomacular adhesion, 74, 74f
vitreomacular traction, 74, 75f, 76f

vitreoretinal lymphoma, 234, 235f, 236f
vitreous, 26, 26f
  opacities in, 31, 32f
vitritis, 170, 175f, 189f, 193f, 198f, 200
Vogt–Koyanagi–Harada disease, 182, 183f
volume scans, 5t
  optic nerve, 38
von Hippel–Lindau disease, 228

W

waterfall effect, 178, 179f, 180f
wet age-related macular degeneration, 46, 47f, 48f, 49f, 50f, 51f, 52f, 53f, 54f
widefield scans, 5t, 6

X

X-linked juvenile retinoschisis, 116, 116f, 117f, 118f

Z

Zeiss Cirrus SD-OCT, 4–6, 5t, 8

Index